Atefeh Asadi Rizi

Stem Cells

AF302625

Atefeh Asadi Rizi

Stem Cells

Noor Publishing

Imprint
Any brand names and product names mentioned in this book are subject to trademark, brand or patent protection and are trademarks or registered trademarks of their respective holders. The use of brand names, product names, common names, trade names, product descriptions etc. even without a particular marking in this work is in no way to be construed to mean that such names may be regarded as unrestricted in respect of trademark and brand protection legislation and could thus be used by anyone.

Cover image: www.ingimage.com

Publisher:
Noor Publishing
is a trademark of
Dodo Books Indian Ocean Ltd. and OmniScriptum S.R.L publishing group

120 High Road, East Finchley, London, N2 9ED, United Kingdom
Str. Armeneasca 28/1, office 1, Chisinau MD-2012, Republic of Moldova, Europe
Printed at: see last page
ISBN: 978-620-5-63460-8

Stem Cells

By

Atefeh Asadi Rizi

Young Researchers and Elite Club, Falavarjan Branch, Islamic Azad University, Isfahan, Iran

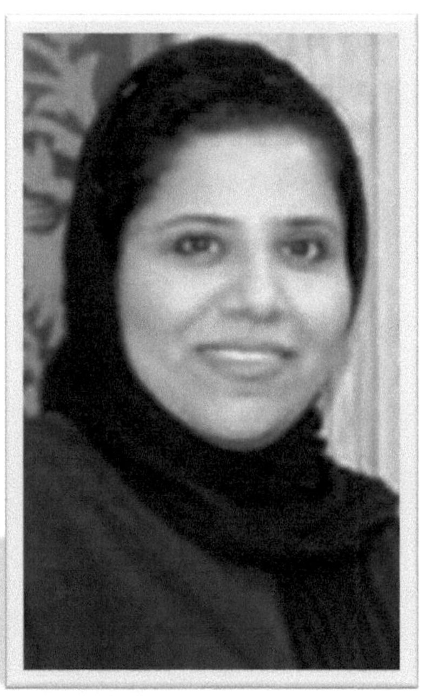

Atefeh Asadi Rizi

Young Researchers and Elite Club, Falavarjan Branch, Islamic Azad University, Isfahan, Iran

Dedicated to the merciful angels who:

The pure moments of believing, enjoying pleasure and pride, seeking courage, achieving greatness and all the unique and beautiful experiences of my life, are due to their green presence.

Dedicated to my dear family, my constant companions, I hope my efforts will help the all communities.

Content

Chapter I

Generalities of the research

Introduction

Stem cells are the raw materials of the body. Cells from which all other cells with special functions are produced. These cells have many applications in the treatment of many diseases. Due to the unique ability of stem cells, these cells are one of the most attractive topics in biology and medical sciences today. Also, research in this field has increased our knowledge about how an organ grows and develops from a single cell, and more importantly, it has helped to understand the mechanism of replacement of healthy cells with damaged cells. In the following, we want to examine the effect of stem cells on a number of diseases.

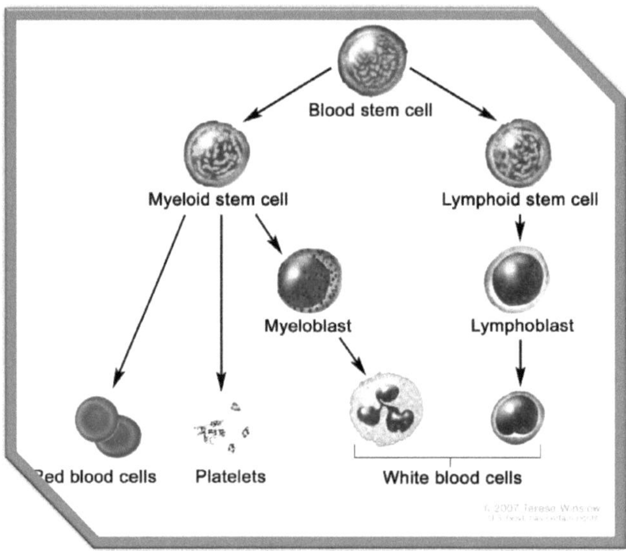

Figure 1. What is a stem cell?

How are stem cells defined?

As mentioned, these cells are the basic materials of the body. These cells divide under suitable conditions in the body or in the laboratory and form more cells called daughter cells. Daughter cells either become new stem cells (self-renewal) or become specialized cells (differentiation) with a more specialized function, such as blood cells, brain cells, heart muscle cells, or bone cells. No other cell in the body has the natural ability to produce new cells. Of course, these cells are not only used to make replacement nerve cells for transplantation. They can be used in other ways, especially as a support for the patient's cells and a controlling or regulating effect on the patient's central nervous system.

In fact, many believe that some stem cells (for example, mesenchymal cells) are uniquely useful in disease. For example, in MS, stem cell transplantation may produce substances that support the survival or recovery of damaged nerve cells. They are also effective in this disease by reducing inflammation. This may prove a valuable approach, regardless of the ability of such cells to become replacement neurons. Likewise, much work has been done with cells of this type in the laboratory. A number of well-powered and well-designed studies have been conducted in small numbers of patients to demonstrate that the procedure is feasible and well tolerated.

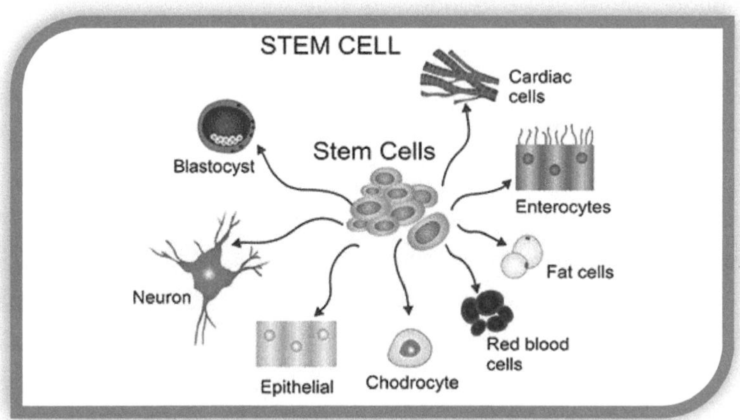

Figure 2. What are Stem Cell Receptors- CUSABIO

Special feature of stem cells

Stem cells are cells that have not yet differentiated. This means that they have not yet been assigned a specific function in the body. At first glance, stem cells are little different from normal body cells. However, they have two very special talents: They can divide and differentiate. So, they can create exact copies of themselves. In addition, they can be defined in a specific cell, thus forming or repairing the tissue.

Types of stem cells

Researchers classify stem cells based on their differentiation potential into other cells. Embryonic cells are the strongest type. Because their task is to become any type of cell in the body. The complete classification includes the following:

- **Competent:** This type of cells can differentiate into possible cell types. The first few cells that appear when the zygote begins to divide are viable.
- **Multipotent:** These cells can become almost any type of cell in the body. Early embryonic cells are multipotent.
- **Multipotent:** These cells can differentiate into a family of closely related cells. For example, adult hematopoietic stem cells can become red or white cells or platelets.
- **Oligopotent:** These can differentiate into several different cell types. Adult lymphoid or myeloid cells can do this.
- **Unototent:** These can only produce cells of one type, which is their own type. However, they are still stem cells because they can renew themselves. For example, we can refer to muscle cells in adults. Embryonic cells are considered pluripotent rather than pluripotent because they cannot become part of the extraembryonic membranes or mate.

The effect of stem cells on spinal cord lesions

Currently, post-accident care for spinal cord injury patients focuses on extensive physical therapy, occupational therapy, and other rehabilitation therapies. A number of published articles and case studies confirm the possibility of treating spinal cord injury with stem cells derived from human umbilical cord tissue and cells derived from bone marrow.

The possibility of combined allogeneic stem cell therapy for spinal cord injury

Many articles and studies have examined and confirmed the effect of this case. This treatment has resulted in improvement in the following cases:

➢ Improve your ASIA score;

➢ Improving bladder or bowel function;

➢ Improve sexual performance;

➢ Increased muscle control.

Through the administration of mesenchymal stem cells derived from umbilical cord tissue, we have observed improvements in spinal cord injury patients treated at our centers.

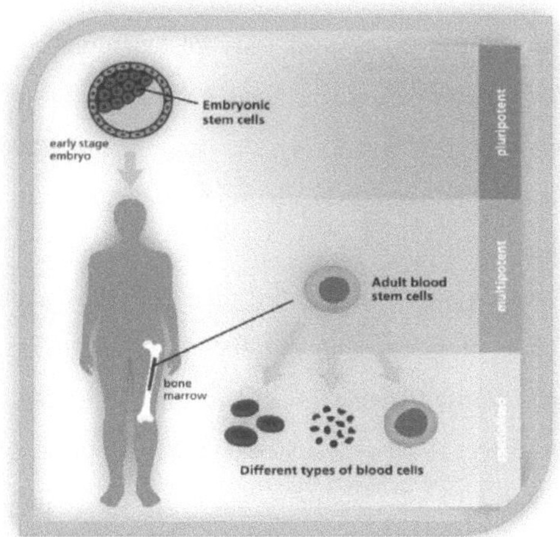

Figure 3. What is a stem cell?

9

Very complex spinal cord injuries

Inflammation occurs, nerve tissue is destroyed, and wounds are created that prevent the growth of nerve cells. Stem cells can help solve all these problems. They can replace dead tissue, produce new nerve cells and create a regenerative environment.

The effect of stem cells on neurological diseases

These cells can be used in the treatment of various diseases of the nervous system, such as stroke, Huntington's disease, Parkinson's disease, lateral sclerosis, amyotrophic, multiple sclerosis and Alzheimer's disease.

MS

Although the underlying cellular and molecular mechanisms of stem cell therapy in patients with MS are not understood, the results have been encouraging. For example, by intravenous injection, mesenchymal cells are able to move in brain lesions and improve the survival rate of brain cells. Also, the injection of mesenchymal cells reduces the severity of the disease and improves the quality of life of MS patients.

These cells can be easily isolated from various body sources, including blood, adipose tissue and bone marrow, umbilical cord blood and placenta. Many studies have analyzed the safety and efficacy of tests related to cells derived from these different sources. The injection of mesenchymal cells derived from bone marrow has been revealed to improve the severity of the disease, the cognitive functions of patients and the quality of life due to the neuroprotective and anti-inflammatory properties of the cells.

Studies have shown that adipose-derived MSC therapy is a safe method that improves MS disabilities, such as problems with sex and social activities. Researchers have determined that adult adipose tissue stem cells are one of the most suitable cells for treating MS. This is because adipose tissue is easily separated, produces a high volume of cells per unit area, and has relatively cheap extraction costs. In addition, umbilical cord-derived mesenchymal cells are attractive therapeutic options because they are derived from an easily accessible tissue and there are no ethical dilemmas. In recent research, it has been determined that hematopoietic stem cell transplantation can prevent the progression of MS disease for 4 to 5 years in 70% to 80% of patients.

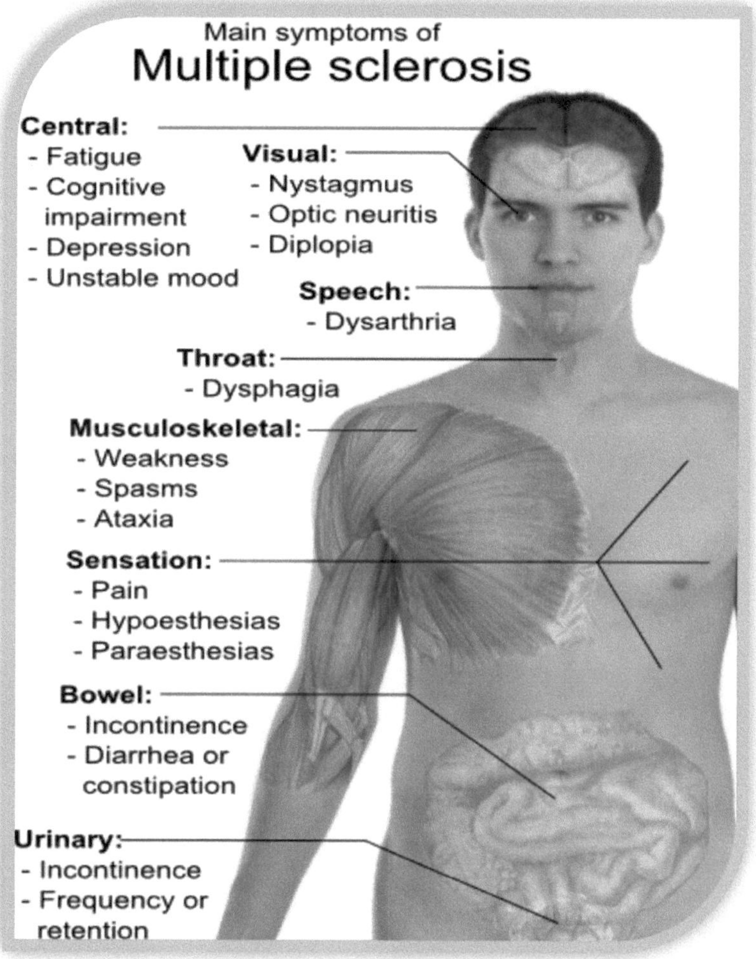

Figure 4. Multiple Sclerosis (MS)

The effect of stem cells on Parkinson's disease

In recent years, research has been conducted on the use of nerve cells derived from aborted human embryos. Obviously, the cell source for treating the disease in this way is very limited and brings many problems. Meanwhile, a suitable and effective alternative for Parkinson's disease cell therapy is dopaminergic progenitor cells derived from fetal cells, which can function as a renewable resource with high capacity, and this method is being researched.

The effect of stem cells on Huntington's disease

Huntington's symptoms include a severe decrease in muscle control, emotional disturbance, and interference in brain cells. This disease is related to the cranial nerve and provides an excellent model for cell replacement therapy. Most of the diseases related to the cranial nerves are currently incurable and often the treatments that are able to affect the main pathogenic factors need a lot of time. This brings into focus strategies such as cell replacement therapy. For this reason, in the last two decades, there has been a great interest in the treatment of neurodegenerative diseases such as Huntington's disease with the method of cell replacement.

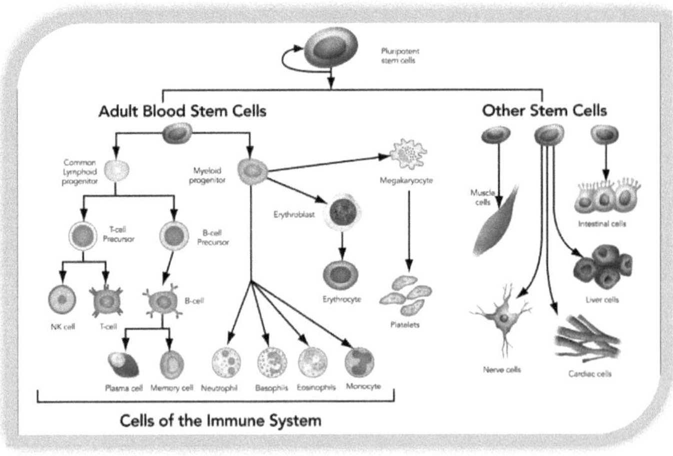

Figure 5. What are Stem Cells?

Are stem cells effective?

According to current research, the effect of using these cells can cure 70 types of diseases in the future.

How much does the treatment cost?

In the city of Tehran, without conducting tests, they are 3 million and 700 thousand tomans with the tests of 4 million 100 thousand tomans. And 160 thousand tomans will be charged as an annual charge after the second year.

Importance of cell banking

Stem cell banking is very important and has the following benefits

> Keeping the cell for a long time without significant change.

> Possible decrease and increase in detection of cell contamination (microbial and cell junction).

> Reducing the costs of cell implantation.

Problems of using stem cells

There are several obstacles to using these cells for treatment. Because it is very difficult to detect and identify stem cells, especially for adults. Also, the responses of the body's immune system can reduce its usefulness. The use of these cells can cause cancer, poisoning, infection, reduced immunity and even death. For this reason, this method should be used when other treatments have not worked. The most powerful include powerful embryonic stem cells as well as induced cells that have the ability to divide, multiply and transform into different types of cells. This power is also their greatest weakness. After being injected into the human body, the cells can begin to multiply uncontrollably which, as a result, potentially cause the growth of tumors.

How to do the process?

The cord blood sample collected after entering the cord blood bank is checked by the quality control unit, and if permission is obtained, it will be processed in the laboratory. The sample is first evaluated in terms of volume and number of cells, and in the next step, if the necessary conditions are met, it enters the process of cell separation. Otherwise, the contract will be canceled by notifying the family and the cost will be returned according to the contract. Microbial and viral tests are carried out on the samples that meet the minimum standard conditions. Finally, it is stored for a long time in special freezing tanks at a temperature of minus 196 degrees Celsius. The frozen sample is used only once for transplantation.

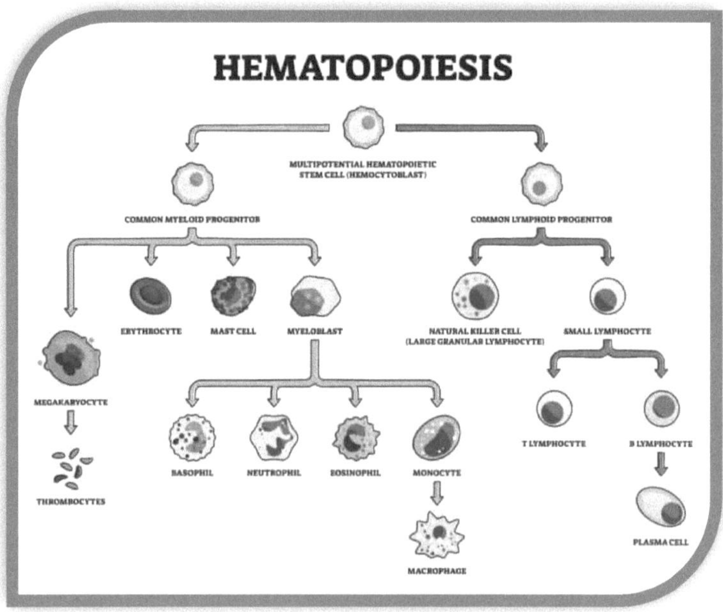

Figure 6. Scientists closer to making blood stem cells in the lab

How do induced pluripotent stem cells produce?

By changing some genes, the signals in the body tell the cell that some genes are on and some genes are off. Scientists re-introduce the signals that remain in the early embryo as stem cells to produce the resulting competent stem cells. These turn off the genes that tell the cell to specialize and turn on the genes that tell the cell to be basal.

What are the limitations of these treatment methods?

Many people have a moral problem with using human embryos for scientific study. Also, the ability of embryonic stem cells to reproduce endlessly means that they may develop mutations that can interfere with their development or allow them to divide to the point where they cause damage. Finding suitable medical applications for embryonic cells is challenging.

Stem cells; Its sources and types and use

Returning to the beginnings and roots is the solution to many of humanity's problems today. In the field of current incurable diseases, an effort is being made to return to these beginnings so that a suitable treatment may be found. Returning to the first cells that turn into other types of cells at the beginning of creation during pregnancy and even trying to go beyond these cells means returning to the genetic language of four or five letters that these cells and all life is made of and genetic measures and interventions in the form of genetic engineering and even the production of vaccines from the language of genes, such as some recent vaccines in the prevention of covid-19 syndrome, are wise efforts that, although we are at the beginning, promise to solve many problems in the history of mankind. It will be special for the treatment of many incurable congenital diseases and neurological diseases.

Each cell in the body performs a specific task, but stem cells do not have a specific role and can later transform into any other cell. Stem cells are undifferentiated cells and can turn into any other cell. The attention of scientists and doctors to stem cells is due to its help in explaining some functions of the body and why sometimes the organs are unable to perform their functions. Scientists are trying to use stem cells to treat some diseases that have no proper treatment today.

Source of stem cells

These cells are obtained from two sources:

1- Cells of adult tissues and fetal body tissues.

2- Scientists try to obtain these cells from other types of cells.

Adult stem cells: The adult human body has a large number of stem cells throughout its life and can use them wherever it is needed. These cells are called somatic stem cells, and they are found in the body from the moment the embryo begins to develop; Although these cells are indeterminate and they are more specialized than embryonic stem cells. The body rebuilds its tissues every day; In some parts of the body, such as viscera and bone marrow, stem cells divide continuously to produce new tissues and maintain them and rebuild them when they are destroyed. Stem cells are found in various tissues.

- ❖ Brain;
- ❖ Bone marrow;
- ❖ Blood and blood vessels;
- ❖ Muscle tissue;
- ❖ Skin;
- ❖ Liver.

But creating stem cells is a difficult task and these cells may remain undifferentiated for years and not divide; As long as the body uses it to repair or regenerate the organ. Stem cells can divide and regenerate themselves endlessly, which means they can make all kinds of organ cells or even regenerate the whole organ. We see that the division and regeneration of these cells explains how to heal skin wounds and how to repair some organs such as the liver; In the past, scientists believed that adult stem cells are differentiated into other types of cells only based on the original tissue in which they are formed. But some reasons show that these cells can differentiate into other types of cells.

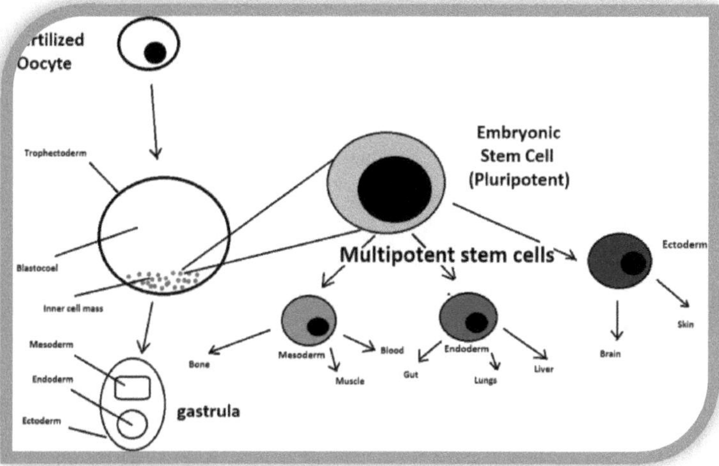

Figure 7. Stem cells: past, present, and future

Embryonic stem cells

From the first stages of pregnancy and after 3 to 5 days from conception, the embryo takes the form of a bag called a blastocyst or a spherical mass of cells that later adheres to the wall of the uterus and this bag is made up of stem cells. Embryonic stem cells come from the blastocyst sac with a life of 4 to 5 days. In laboratory pregnancy or IVF, scientists grow several egg cells in a test tube so that at least one of them can survive and grow; When the sperm fertilizes the egg, these two cells turn into a single cell called a zygote (fertilized egg); Then the zygote divides and two, four, eight, etc. cells are formed; until the fetus is formed. Before replacing this mass in the uterus, it consists of 150-200 cells called blastocysts.

This bag consists of two parts

The inner cell mass that becomes part of the placenta.

The external cell mass that becomes part of the human body.

We see embryonic stem cells in the inner cell mass and scientists call it stem cells with full strength. This expression indicates that these cells have the ability to differentiate into any other cells in the body, and in the presence of sufficient stimulation, these cells can turn into blood cells or skin cells or any other type of cells in the body. In the early stages of pregnancy, the blastocyst sac exists for 5 days - before the embryo is implanted in the uterus - and at this stage, the stem cells begin to differentiate and the embryonic stem cells turn into various types of cells, including adult stem cells.

Interstitial stem cells (mesenchymal)

Interstitial stem cells are developing tissues. This tissue is a curtain that surrounds body organs and other tissues, and scientists use interstitial stem cells to produce other tissues such as bone, cartilage, and fat cells, and these cells are used very vitally today.

Stimulated stem cells with great power

Scientists have produced these cells in the laboratory using skin cells and specific cells from other tissues, and these cells are used in the same way as embryonic stem cells, and in this way, they are useful in the treatment of many diseases. But it still needs a lot of research work for improvement. To produce stem cells, scientists first remove samples from adult or fetal tissues, then place these cells in a special environment so that these cells multiply; But they will never differentiate. Scientists use stem cells for specific purposes and can differentiate these cells in a specific way, and this method is called direct differentiation. To date, producing large numbers of embryonic stem cells is easier than producing adult stem cells, but scientists have made progress in both cases.

Types of stem cells

Scientists have divided stem cells into several categories based on the power of reproduction, differentiation and production of other types of cells, and embryonic stem cells have the most power and can produce all types of cells.

1- Cells with full strength: These cells can be differentiated into different types of cells; Such as a zygote cell or an egg.

2- Cells with high power: These cells can be transformed into almost any other cell. For example, the cells in the early embryonic stages are of this type.

3- Cells with multiple powers: These cells can be transformed into different types of cells of the same type. For example, mature stem cells that are formed for blood can be transformed into white and red blood cells of some other blood components.

4- Low power cells: These cells can become a small number of cells such as lymphoid cells and brain cells.

5- Cells with only one power: It produces only one type of cells, but it is classified as stem cells, but it can regenerate itself like stem cells. Adult muscle cells, which are embryonic stem cells with a lot of power, because they cannot differentiate.

Application of stem cells

Stem cells, in turn, do not fulfill a specific purpose, but they are important in several aspects, and despite proper stimulation, they can produce any cell, that is, they can regenerate damaged tissues under certain conditions, and they can regenerate organs or repairing the tissues and rebuilding the lost tissues.

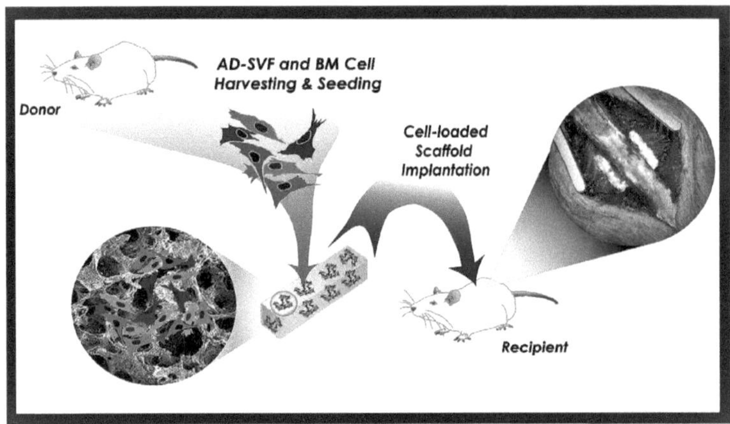

Figure 8. Research Story Tip: Johns Hopkins Medicine Puts Fat to Good Use as Stem Cell Source for Spinal Fusion Surgery

Tissue regeneration: This regeneration is one of the most important uses of stem cells, but until today, if a patient needs a new tissue such as a kidney, he must wait for a person to donate a kidney; Scientists can use stem cells and by stimulating them and growing them in a certain way, they can produce certain organs. For example, doctors use the stem cells under the human skin to create new skin tissue and have been able to treat burns and other skin injuries by replacing this tissue with the lost tissue. The title of orthokine therapy is a new method in the treatment of arthritis of the joints, an attempt to treat spinal cord injury, the injection of mesenchymal stem cells (MSCs) in the treatment of stroke patients, and those with autism and cerebral palsy will be treated with stem cells in the not-too-distant future. Scientists produce heart stem cells.

Researches and scientific discoveries: Stem cells are not only useful in treatment but also used in scientific researchers. For example, scientists have realized that removing a certain gene or adding it causes the differentiation of these cells, and this knowledge helps to identify any gene or mutation that has caused a specific effect. By this means, scientists have been able to discover the cause of many diseases, many of which have not yet had a cure. The abnormal division and differentiation of cells leads to cancer and mood disorders that we have seen since childhood, and knowing what causes the abnormal division and differentiation of these cells helps to treat these diseases. Also, stem cells have led to the development of some treatments, and instead of testing these drugs on healthy and sick people to determine their usefulness, scientists can test these treatments on tissues made from stem cells.

Treatment with stem cells and drug and medicine organization

Some people try to use stem cells for specific purposes in treatment, including preventing aging, and yet many of these uses have not been approved by the food and drug administration, and some are illegal and dangerous, and anyone who wants to use of stem cells in the treatment of diseases must be approved by the food and drug administration.

What are stem cells and why are they so important?

Stem cells have a significant ability to differentiate into all types of body cells. In addition, in many tissues, they are used as an internal tissue repair system. In fact, stem cells have two key characteristics that distinguish them from other cells.

> ➤ Self-renewal;
> ➤ Differentiation.

Self-regeneration

Self- regeneration means that the stem cell is able to reproduce itself for a long time. This sentence means that these cells have the ability to reproduce and divide continuously and have no limitations in this regard. It should be noted that in some organs, such as the intestine and bone marrow, stem cells divide regularly to repair and replace worn out or damaged tissues, but in other organs, such as the pancreas and heart, stem cells divide only under certain conditions.

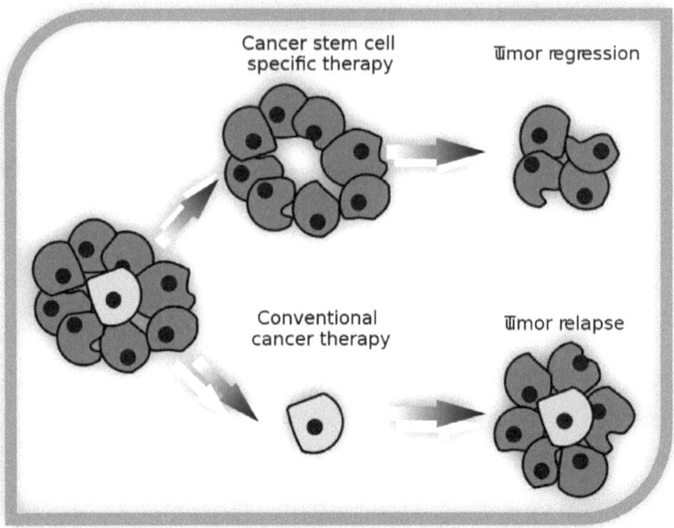

Figure 9. Cancer stem cell

Distinction

Having this feature in the stem cell enables it to transform into differentiated cells with a specific function under special conditions in the body or laboratory environment. Stem cells are important to living organisms for many reasons. In general, stem cells are divided into three categories based on their characteristics:

➢ Embryonic stem cells;

➢ Mature stem cells;

➢ Umbilical cord stem cells.

In the 3 to 5-day old embryo, which is called blastocyst (Blastocystis), internal cells create the whole body of the living organism including all types of specialized cells and different organs such as heart, lung, skin, sperm, zygote and other tissues. The inner mass of blastocyst cells is the main source of embryonic stem cells. In some mature tissues such as bone marrow, muscles and brain, there are also discrete populations of mature stem cells whose task is to repair or replace damaged cells.

Due to their unique regenerative abilities, stem cells offer a new potential to treat diseases such as diabetes and heart diseases, which, of course, require many tests to enter the clinical field. Stem cell research also advances knowledge about how an organ develops from a single cell, and healthy cells replace damaged cells in mature organs. Research on stem cells is one of the most interesting parts of modern biology, which, like many expanded fields in scientific research, raises questions and challenges that will lead to new discoveries in the future.

Features of stem cells

All stem cells, regardless of origin, have three general characteristics that distinguish them from other cells.

> ➢ They are able to divide and regenerate for long periods of time.
> ➢ Cells are not specialized.
> ➢ They can differentiate into specific cells.

Based on differentiation and reversibility, stem cells can be divided into the following three parts:

1- Totipotent

This category is able to make all cells (single cells and paired cells), which makes them ideal for cell and gene therapy, as well as tissue engineering for transplantation and replacement of diseased cells. This means that the therapeutic value of pluripotent stem cells is very high. By learning about the process of division, we can overcome the process of disease development and then come up with ways to prevent the production and division of diseased cells.

2- Pluripotent stem cells

These cells have the ability to differentiate into most specialized cells of the body. They are another type of stem cell that can make most or all of a person's cells. For example, the embryonic stem cell under certain conditions can make a person, but it is not able to make a placenta. The cells obtained from the fetal gonads are called embryonic germ cells, which are also part of the omnipotence category. Each of these cells has the ability to create a colony and forms the three embryonic layers by differentiation.

3- Multipotent stem cells

Like other stem cells, they have the main characteristics, but they create a limited number of cells and the happy ones also have a smaller number than others. Examples of pluripotent stem cells are cells that are in the brain and create different nerve cells and neuroglia cells (supporting cells of the nervous system) that can create all kinds of blood cells but cannot create brain cells. Bone marrow also contains pluripotent stem cells that cause the creation of various types of blood cells (globules).

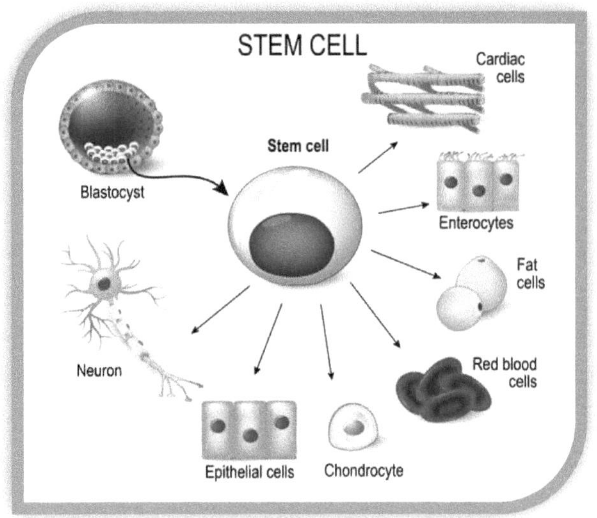

Figure 10. Stem Cell Therapy for Alzheimer's

Chapter II
Application of stem cells

Stem cells taken from the umbilical cord are special. They are young, strong and dynamic, and numerous clinical studies have been conducted on them around the world, which confirmed the suitability of these cells in the regeneration of damaged tissue after the events of reducing degenerative diseases such as intervertebral disc and cancer treatment. Many experts and scientists believe about the potential of stem cells that these cells will play a very important role in the treatment of diseases in the next few decades.

Treatment of spinal cord injuries

So far, from many cells and tissues such as stem cells, olfactory sheath cells, (cells that produce myelin on the surface of the olfactory nerves), Schwann cells, (cells that produce myelin on the surface of the peripheral nerves), the root of the dorsal ganglion, the tissue of the above gland. Kidney and transgenic cells have been used as cell sources in the treatment of spinal cord injuries.

Cell transplantation after spinal cord injuries is done for several purposes
- Creating a connection between the two sides of the lesion;
- replacing dead cells in order to create new neurons or oligodendrocytes;
- Providing the right environment to induce restoration.

Among the first pioneers of using these cells in the topic of cell therapy and spinal lesions were McDonald and his colleagues in 1999. Their studies showed that the transplantation of mouse embryonic stem cells to rats with spinal cord injury improves the performance and behavior of rats. The histological results showed the differentiation of these cells into astrocytes, oligodendrocytes and neurons during the next 2 to 5 weeks and their migration to 8 mm away from the lesion area. Neural progenitors derived from stem cells produce significant amounts of laminin and fibronectin, both of which are factors that promote the survival of nerve cells and can be effective in wound healing. According to McDonald's results, one of the important issues in the discussion of spinal cord lesions is the loss of myelin and the subsequent loss of physiological and behavioral functions of the cells in the central nervous system.

Therefore, the remyelination of healthy axons without myelination is considered an important regenerative role in the treatment of spinal cord injuries. In this regard, some believe that the ability to differentiate embryonic stem cells into a pure population of oligodendrocyte precursors is of special importance in clinical applications. Currently, through the administration of mesenchymal stem cells derived from the umbilical cord tissue, improvement has been observed in patients with spinal cord injuries, and thus the improvement of spinal cord diseases is also one of the other applications of stem cells.

The role of stem cells in burn healing

Zed Merrick, a 2-year-old child who had 2nd degree burns, was completely cured by spraying healthy tissue cells and cell proliferation!! One of the uses of stem cells is their role in healing burns and accelerating the healing of wounds. The skin is a very complex tissue that accounts for about 10% of the body mass. For this reason, its burn has significant consequences on human physical and mental health. At present, there is no artificial skin that is completely designed and has the ability to be transplanted on the damaged skin, and only surgery has solved this problem to some extent, which also solves problems such as uneven skin color, scars, and other cosmetic and even movement defects. Combined treatment using stem cells and tissue matrix. The meaning of cell therapy in the treatment of burns is to replace damaged tissues with healthy cells cultured in the laboratory. Then, after about 3 to 5 weeks, these cultured cells are injected into the burned areas by a carrier and create an epidermis-like covering on the damaged surface. Using this method, granulation (excess flesh on the burn site) will also not occur.

Leukemia (blood cancer)

Comparison of blood cells of a healthy person and a person with leukemia

In leukemia, some cells of the hematopoietic system get out of control and start dividing uncontrollably. As the disease worsens, these cells attack other body tissues and disrupt their function. Doctors currently use chemotherapy and radiation methods to control this disease, but this treatment also kills other normal cells. Therefore, it has many side effects, but stem cells have different functions to treat this disease. Some strengthen the immune system in a specific way and others cause cancer cells to be better identified by the immune system.

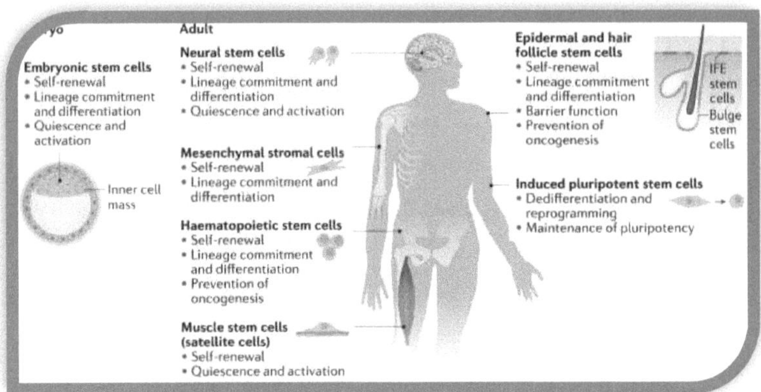

Figure 11. Translational control of stem cell function | Nature Reviews Molecular Cell Biology

Using cells against cells

Scientific and technological advances in recent years, especially in the field of stem cells, have caused the treatment of cancer patients to experience new dimensions. The use of immune cells to treat brain tumors will increase the glimmers of hope for treatment in these patients and other cancer sufferers. This work was started by domestic universities and knowledge-based companies, and the technology of isolation and activation of immune cells was obtained by the country's technologists. With this technology, it became possible to target brain tumor cells in the laboratory environment as well as pre-clinical models.

Diseases that can be treated with stem cells. Umbilical cord blood stem cells are used in the treatment of more than 100 diseases. A list of diseases that can be treated using umbilical cord blood stem cells is as follows:

- **Stem cell disorders:** Aplastic anemia, Fanconi anemia, paroxysmal nocturnal hemoglobinuria (PNH);
- **Acute leukemia:** AML, ALL, acute undifferentiated leukemia;
- **Chronic leukemia:** CML;
- **Diseases of defects in the production of lymphocytes:** Non-Hodgkin's lymphoma, Hodgkin's lymphoma;
- **Hereditary abnormalities of red blood cells:** Beta, thalassemia major, sickle cell anemia;
- **Congenital immune system disorders:** Costman's syndrome, leukocyte adhesion defect, D. George's syndrome;
- **Hereditary platelet defects:** Congenital thrombocytopenia;
- **Plasma cell disorders:** Multiple myeloma, plasma cell leukemia;
- **Hereditary diseases:** Lash Nyhan syndrome, cartilage hypoplasia;
- **Other diseases:** Alzheimer's disease, diabetes, Parkinson's, spinal injuries, heart and brain strokes, liver diseases, muscular dystrophy.

The perspective of using stem cells

Today, it has been proven that stem cells are capable of treating a wide range of chronic and acute diseases, and a lot of research is being done in the field of using stem cells in the treatment of diseases such as Parkinson's, heart disease, liver disease, diabetes, muscular dystrophy, spinal cord injuries, and stroke. done

- **Alzheimer's:** 1 out of 10 people over the age of 65 and 5 out of 10 people over the age of 85 suffer from this disease.

- ➢ **Spinal cord injuries:** Spinal cord injuries affect more than 750,000 people in the United States each year.
- ➢ **Bone regeneration:** Hope for the treatment of patients with Parkinson's osteoporosis.
- ➢ **MS:** It is an autoimmune and progressive disease related to the central nervous system that affects many people every year.

Persistence of cells after storage

According to the international standards of the AABB and Fact Net Cord umbilical cord blood banks, which the Royan umbilical cord blood bank also operates based on these standards, they have announced the preservation of samples for up to 25 years. This number does not mean that cells cannot be used after 25 years. Because the coldness of the cells is provided by nitrogen and they are kept at minus 196 degrees Celsius. At this temperature, all the activities of the cell stop and it seems that it is possible to maintain the cell in these conditions without restrictions. Of course, to prove this theory, after 25 years, these cells will be tested for their vital capabilities.

Cancer

Inactivation of "Cancer stem cells" (CSCs) is crucial for tumor treatment after radiation therapy. Cancer stem cells are tumor cells that have unlimited cell division and the ability to reassemble the entire tumor. These cells play a central role in tumor growth, progression and recurrence after treatment. This definition means that stem cancer cells must be disabled to permanently eradicate the tumor. Because of their importance in tumor treatment, stem cancer cells can be used to optimize anticancer treatments.

Diabetes

The most common cause of diabetes is the inability to make enough insulin. Successful strategies to treat diabetes must restore the function of pancreatic beta cells destroyed by the immune system and overcome the destruction of insulin-producing cells. Recent studies have shown that with the help of stem cells, insulin production can be increased in patients suffering from diabetes. Researchers have tried to transform human stem cells into insulin-producing cells that can be transplanted into diabetic patients. This work will pave the way for effective novel diabetes cells.

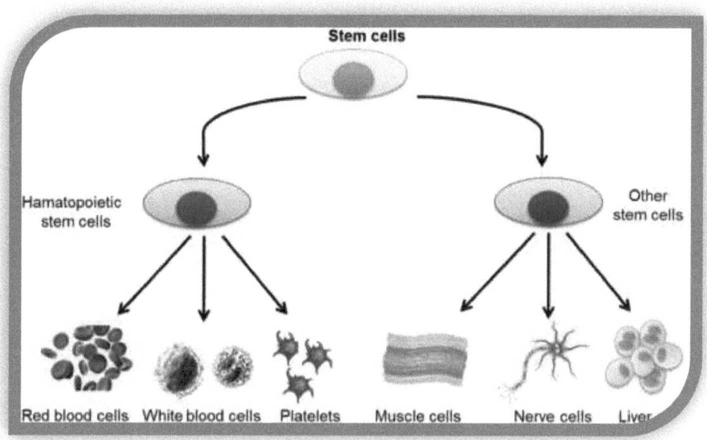

Figure 12. Stem Cells - an overview

Parkinson

"Parkinson's disease" (PD) is tremor at rest, which is more common in old age but can also be seen in young people. This disease occurs due to the destruction of cells that secrete a substance called dopamine (which is a neurotransmitter). Parkinson's disease destroys the neurons that produce the dopamine transporter, which causes movement disorders in people. Recent research shows that it is possible to transplant neural stem cells from the central nervous system against inflammatory damage to the mechanism of this part. Treatment using stem cells, if proven, will be one of the successful methods for treating Parkinson's disease.

Huntington's disease

"Huntington's disease" (HD) is caused by a mutation in the gene encoding Huntington's protein. The symptoms of Huntington's disease include a severe decrease in muscle control, emotional disturbance, and pathological interactions (pathology) in brain cells. This disease is related to the cranial nerve and provides an excellent model for cell replacement therapy. Most neurodegenerative diseases are currently incurable, and treatments that are able to target the underlying pathogens often require a long time. This issue focuses on strategies such as cell replacement therapy. For this reason, in the last two decades, there has been a lot of interest in the treatment of Huntington's disease with the method of cell replacement.

Advantages and disadvantages of using stem cells

The safety and efficacy of using stem cells obtained from blood or bone marrow for the regeneration of hematopoietic stem cells have been proven. In addition, hematopoietic stem cells and stem cells obtained from sources such as adipose tissue are used to treat orthopedic, neurological and other diseases. Despite the lack of evidence from controlled clinical trials, some doctors believe that stem cells have a unique capacity to restore health because these cells can sense their surroundings and act in such a way as to correct any ailment. Another theory is that conducting controlled trials and regular standards for such promising treatments is too complicated for all industry sponsors; Therefore, extensive use of these cells in clinical trials is needed. Proponents of both theories believe that treatment using stem cells is relatively safe. The theory that stem cells are inherently able to sense the environment they enter and identify areas such as knee cartilage that need repair or replacement is not based on scientific evidence.

Advantages of using cell therapy

Today, the use of tuberculosis therapy is used in the treatment of many diseases and many diseases can be improved by using this type of treatment method. Of course, research on stem cells and how to use them in the treatment of incurable and expensive diseases is still ongoing, and in the coming years we will see the development of this type of treatment. To perform tuberculosis therapy, it is necessary to take samples of stem cells so that they can be cultured in a laboratory environment and transformed into the desired cells for the treatment of the disease using genetic changes. Stem cells are naturally present in every person's body and there is a special type of them in every area and organ. These cells work naturally in the body and are responsible for repairing damaged tissues and dead cells and are effective in delaying aging. But with the help of cell therapy science, stem cells can be modified and strengthened to be effective in the treatment of various diseases. Among the benefits of using stem cells and treatment using tuberculosis therapy, the following can be mentioned:

- The fields of regenerative medicine and cloning therapy;
- Treatment of diseases such as cancer, schizophrenia, Alzheimer's disease, Parkinson's disease, spinal injuries and diabetes;
- Growth of cells of organs and vital organs of the body using stem cells and their transplantation in the patient's body;
- Contributing to medical research regarding the growth of fetal cells and preventing aging and death;
- Making all kinds of medicines needed to treat certain diseases using cell therapy;
- Examining all types of drugs on stem cell samples for therapeutic analysis and analysis and identifying their possible side effects and problems;
- Conducting research to identify natural ways to prevent aging and achieve long life;
- Discovering new ways to delay cell erosion;

- ➢ High probability of acceptance of the body's immune system in the use of stem cells harvested from the patient's body;
- ➢ Using tuberculosis therapy in order to delay the activity of destructive and mutated cells;
- ➢ Artificial fertilization and the birth of laboratory embryos to extract embryonic stem cells and test various genetic and cell therapy methods on them;
- ➢ Research to discover ways to prevent abnormal births and reduce organ defects in babies;
- ➢ Reducing the probability of the birth of a fetus with congenital diseases;
- ➢ Transforming stem cells into the types of cells needed in the body and creating higher flexibility than normal in order to prevent the reoccurrence of disorders.

Disadvantages of using cell therapy

Tuberculosis therapy, like all other treatment methods, has disadvantages and defects that cause various side effects and effects on patients. Among these disadvantages are:

The use of this treatment method can in some cases cause abnormal effects and mutations in the body that are not possible in the normal state. Treatment using stem cells can lead to narrowing of coronary heart vessels. The use of stem cells in the treatment of tuberculosis cannot treat all patients and cure all diseases. According to statistics, only 50% of patients succeed in being treated and accepted by the body's immune system. Destruction of blastocyst cells of eggs due to in vitro fertilization of embryonic stem cells in the body. One of the limitations of cell therapy is that stem cells of any part of the body, such as blood stem cells, are only able to transform into different types of blood cells and cannot be converted into different types of blood cells. used brain cell therapy.

The probability of fetal stem cells not being accepted by the patient's body and by the person's immune system is very high, because these cells were not extracted from the patient's body. There are different treatment methods to treat cancer. One of these methods is cell therapy. In this method, stem cells are injected into the patient's body and replace the damaged cells. This treatment method will have side effects like other methods, but on the other hand, it is one of the effective treatment methods to destroy cancer cells.

Transplant replacement cell therapy

Wake Forest Institute Regenerative Medicine researchers are looking for a promising approach to treat chronic kidney damage and regenerate damaged tissues using stem cells. Kidney diseases are a global problem that can occur chronically and acutely. Using the unique properties of amniotic fluid-derived stem cells, researchers at WFIRM have shown that these cells can potentially restore organ function in a preclinical model of kidney disease. The results of their study have shown that this type of stem cells can be an ideal cell source and a promising therapeutic strategy for patients suffering from chronic and debilitating diseases. Amniotic fluid-derived stem cells have multi lineage differentiation ability as well as anti-inflammatory ability, which makes them a potential cell source for regeneration.

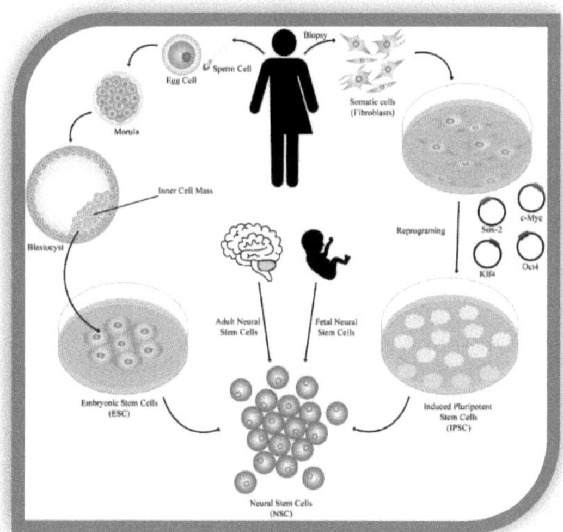

Figure 13. Frontiers, Successes and Hurdles in Stem Cells Application and Production for Brain Transplantation

These cells do not stimulate the immune response, and their use does not lead to tumorigenesis, and they do not bring ethical concerns related to cell sources such as embryonic stem cells. In this study, Dr. Anthony Atala and colleagues at WFIRM found that amniotic fluid stem cells injected into an injured kidney in an animal model led to improved kidney function after 10 weeks. The results of the biopsy showed a decrease in the damage to the capillary clusters (glomerules) in these animals. The results of this study show that treatment with amniotic fluid stem cells has positive effects on the functional improvement and structural recovery of the kidney.

Using cell therapy to treat type 2 diabetes and improve weight

A study has been published in the journal Experimental Biology and Medicine that introduces a new treatment strategy for weight loss and type 2 diabetes. In this study, Dr. Wang and colleagues at Jiao Tong University report that transplantation of MSCs isolated from adipose tissue improves metabolic balance and reduces inflammation in an animal model.

Modern urban lifestyle and inactivity along with diets high in sugar and fat have made diabetes a common problem. Statistics provided by the World Health Organization (WHO) indicate that 90% of the 347 million people in the world with diabetes have type 2 diabetes. In type 2 diabetes, the body cannot use insulin properly, this process is called insulin resistance. Initially, the pancreas produces extra insulin, but over time, it cannot prepare enough insulin, and as a result, the blood sugar level increases. If this condition is not treated, high blood sugar levels will damage organs such as the heart, kidneys, nerves and eyes. Weight gain is a factor involved in the occurrence of type 2 diabetes and inflammation that occurs during the process of weight gain and obesity and increases insulin resistance.

Preliminary clinical studies show that MSC transplantation improves metabolic balance in type 2 diabetes. MSCs isolated from adipose tissue are abundant and easily obtained. However, their ability to improve metabolic function in type 2 diabetes and obesity is not fully understood. In a new study, Dr. Wang and his colleagues evaluated the ability of mesenchymal stem cells isolated from fat to reduce insulin resistance in mice fed a high-fat diet (HFD). Mice fed a high-fat diet that received these cells showed reduced blood sugar levels and improved insulin sensitivity.

More importantly, transplantation of mesenchymal stem cells isolated from adipose that expressed more neuregulin4 had a more effective effect on reducing blood sugar levels and insulin resistance. These beneficial effects appear to be due to suppression of inflammation and enhancement of glucose reabsorption in skeletal muscle and adipose tissue. Overall, this study has shown that transplantation of adipose-isolated MSCs improves glucose tolerance and metabolic balance in high-fat diet-fed mice through multiple mechanisms.

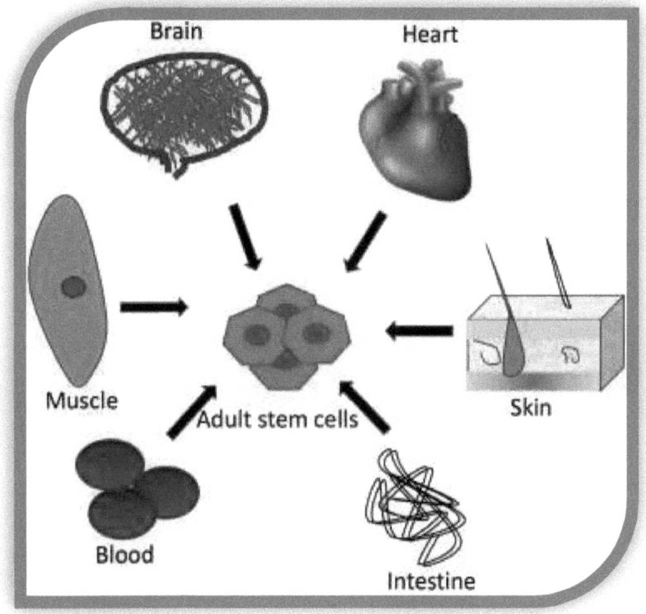

Figure 14. Adult Stem Cell

Stem cell therapy to combat aging

Two small clinical trials have shown that stem cell therapy is safe and completely effective in reversing signs of age-related frailty. In old age, people face a decline in physical performance and immune system. In a study, the physical performance of people before and after six months of stem cell injection was investigated. The tests included activities such as a six-minute walk, a physical performance test, and a breathing test. Also, the researchers tested the participants six months after the blood transfusion to check the immune markers of weakness, and this was in the condition that the participants were given a questionnaire about the quality of sexual intercourse.

In another study, patients with an average age of 76 years had an injection with a high density of human bone marrow mesenchymal stem cells (20 million, 100 million, or 200 million cells) taken from donors between the ages of 20 and 45. Studies have shown no side effects. The researchers found that people who received 100 million cells experienced significant improvement in all of the measured parameters mentioned earlier. The next step in the path of these researches is to conduct larger clinical trials in different places. If stem cell injection is proven to be effective, only a large randomized clinical trial (phase 3) will be needed for public approval so that this method can be used universally in the medical world.

Corona treatment with the help of umbilical cord stem cells

The results of a new study on 24 patients with Covid-19 show that the injection of stem cells from the umbilical cord of newborn babies doubles the possibility of these people recovering. Stem cells from the umbilical cord of newborn babies may be a life-saving treatment for people with severe forms of Covid-19. A study by a group of researchers from the University of Miami in the United States showed that the use of stem cells in patients under 85 years of age doubles the possibility of recovery of these people after contracting Covid-19.

Stem cells treat the respiratory system due to their extraordinary ability to renew and repair damaged tissues. These researchers claim that they can treat 10,000 patients using the cells of an umbilical cord. It acts like a smart technological bomb in the lungs, says Camilo Ricord, the senior researcher of this study. More precisely, this treatment restores the normal immune response and reverses the dangerous complications of the disease. The mentioned research is presented according to the information of 24 patients. These patients suffered from acute respiratory distress syndrome after contracting the corona virus. Each of them was injected with placebo or stem cells twice a day. The recovery rate of the patients in the control group (who received stem cells) was 91% and the patients in the placebo group were 42%. The only person who died despite receiving said treatment was over 85 years old. The researchers also found that patients who received stem cell treatment recovered faster. More than half of them left the hospital within two weeks of receiving the final dose of the drug.

Also, one month after receiving this treatment method, 80% of the control group had no signs of disease. According to Ricordi, two compounds containing 100 million stem cells were injected into each patient within three days. In total, each person in the control group received 200 million stem cells. Also, no side effects due to receiving treatment were observed in the body of the patients. Stem cells have antimicrobial activities that accelerate tissue regeneration, lung and other body organ repair.

Vitiligo treatment with cell therapy

An important disease caused by pigment disorder is vitiligo or leprosy. In this disease, melanocyte cells lose the ability to produce melanin and white spots appear on the skin, and the appearance of these spots is the source of many social and psychological problems. In the cell therapy method, first a small piece of the patient's skin is removed and the melanocyte cells are extracted after interactions and multiplied in a special culture medium. These melanocytes are cultured on a special plate and then created at the site of the wound, and the layer of cultured melanocyte cells is placed on the site of the wound. These cells belong to the individual and do not stimulate the immune system.

The success rate of treatment in this method is between 50% and 70%. This method is used as the last line of treatment in treatment-resistant cases. Another use of the cell therapy method is the use of keratinocyte cell culture at the site of wounds caused by various diseases. Considering that keratinocytes increase during wound healing and cover the surface of the dermis, the use of cultured keratinocytes can act as a barrier to prevent infection, keep the wound moist and accelerate wound healing. Most of the studies conducted by keratinocyte culture in skin wounds have shown an average of 25% to 85% improvement in reducing the size of the wounds. In addition to other necessary measures to care for the burn patient, services are also performed to remove irreversibly burned tissues and close wounds. The establishment of the cell therapy clinic of the skin and stem cell research center is a promise for skin patients and skin rejuvenation applicants.

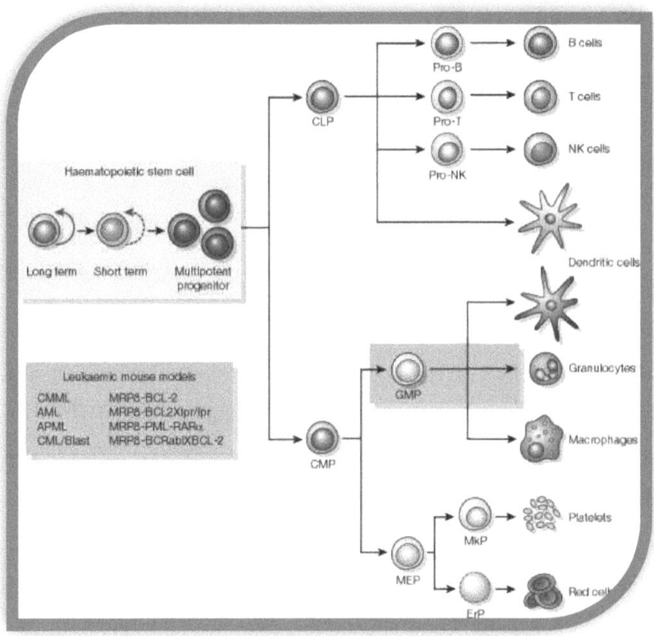

Figure 15. Stem cells, cancer, and cancer stem cells

Embryonic stem cells

Scientists believe that every internal organ of the body has its own stem cells. For example, we can mention blood cells that were made from blood stem cells. However, stem cells appear in the earliest stages of human development, and when scientists grow these cells, they call them embryonic stem cells. The reason why scientists attach great importance to embryonic stem cells is that embryonic stem cells can make any organ or tissue during embryonic development. This means that embryonic stem cells, unlike adult embryonic cells, can become hundreds of other types of cells. For example, as blood stem cells can only make blood cells, embryonic stem cells can make blood, bone, skin, brain, etc.

In addition, stem cells are programmed to make tissues and even organs when mature stem cells cannot do so. This means that embryonic stem cells have a much greater potential to treat diseased organs. Embryonic stem cells were made from embryos left in the laboratory containers after fertility treatments, which did not live more than a few days. If they did not use them, they would throw them away. In fact, scientists take stem cells from embryos. They are usually extra embryos resulting from in vitro or artificial insemination (IVF). In IVF clinics, doctors fertilize several egg cells in a test tube to ensure that at least one of them survives. Then, a limited number of fertilized eggs are replaced in the uterus to start the pregnancy. In fact, the stem cell is the mother of all cells and has the ability to transform into all cells in the body.

These cells have the ability of self-renewing and differentiating into all types of cells, including blood, heart, nerve and cartilage cells. Also, it is effective in the reconstruction and repair of tissues in different parts of the body after damage and injury, and they can be transplanted into the damaged tissues where most of their cells have been lost, replacing the damaged cells, and repairing and repairing defects in that tissue.

Embryonic stem cell function

Due to the unique ability of stem cells, these cells are an attractive topic in biology and medical sciences today. Also, research in this field has increased our knowledge about how an organ grows and develops from a single cell, and more importantly, it has helped to understand the mechanism of replacement of healthy cells with damaged cells. The embryonic stem cell searches inside the body and finds the damaged areas and then tries to repair and treat that part, and at the same time it reproduces, which itself causes the stimulation of the body's repair mechanism.

The treatments performed in that center using the stem cell method are not antigenic and can be applied to any disease without any side effects, rejection, lack of response to drug treatment, or any side effects. When a patient receives fresh embryonic cells, the first action of these cells is to stimulate the cells in the host's system and make them stronger. Then, these cells actually replace the host's immune cells and thus merge with them. This means that they continuously grow more embryonic cells and create a newer and stronger immune system. Cancer treatment with this method makes it possible for chemotherapy and radiation therapy to continue for a longer period of time and actually eliminates their side effects.

In short, stem cells can be described as follows

The human body is made of different types of cells. Many cells are specialized and perform special functions, such as red blood cells that carry oxygen throughout the body in the bloodstream and receive carbon dioxide from the cells. This is while, for example, red blood cells are not able to divide. Stem cells provide the body with new cells as the organism grows and replace the damaged or lost specialized cells. Stem cells have two unique properties that enable them to do this:

> These cells have the ability of successive divisions to produce new cells.
> At the same time that these cells divide, they can differentiate into different and specialized cell types.

In general, stem cell studies are a promising field for the treatment of many diseases for which there is currently no treatment. Unfortunately, in recent years, we have seen a significant growth of types of cancer among different age groups, which affect people's lifestyle and social status. Fortunately, effective treatments for many types of cancer have been identified today. These treatment methods are classified into four general groups, which are: Surgery, hormone-therapy, radiation therapy and chemotherapy.

Chemotherapy

Chemotherapy is a method that is widely used to treat cancer. The term chemotherapy refers to drugs that affect cancer cells and stop them from growing or dividing. This is done by killing dividing cells. The effectiveness of this method depends to some extent on the level and progress of the cancer. Chemotherapy is a drug treatment that uses strong chemicals to kill rapidly growing cells in the body. Chemotherapy is often used to treat cancer because cancer cells grow and multiply much faster than most cells in the body. There are many chemotherapy drugs available that are used alone or in combination to treat a wide variety of cancers.

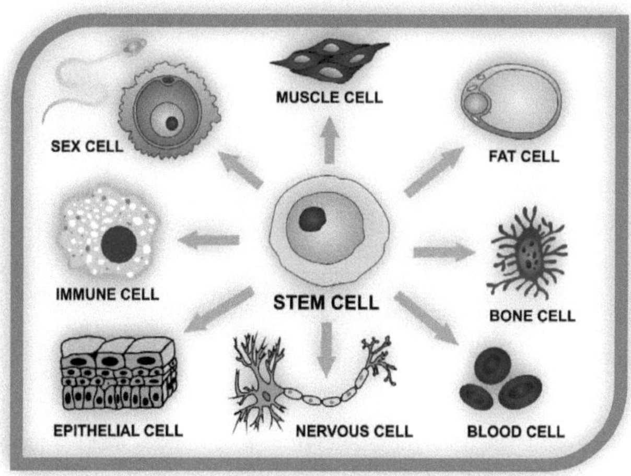

Figure 16. Final stem cell differentiation

Chemotherapy drugs

Chemotherapy drugs are able to destroy cells that have a high growth rate, and by reducing the growth rate and destruction of cancer cells, the symptoms related to cancer will be alleviated quickly.

Chemotherapy affects cancer cells in different ways

- It destroys a part of the cancer cell;
- It stops the growth of cancer cells;
- Cuts off the necessary food for cancer cells.

Different methods of chemotherapy

- Chemotherapy drugs are prescribed in several ways;
- Intramuscular or subcutaneous injection or directly into the cerebrospinal fluid;
- Intravenous injection method that is prescribed through an angioket or through a port in the central veins of the body;
- Intra-arterial injection method in which the chemotherapy drug is usually administered directly in the arteries feeding the tumor;
- Oral method in the form of tablets, capsules or liquid that the patient eats;
- Local or rubbing method where the chemotherapy drug is rubbed on the patient's skin.

In the treatment of breast cancer, intravenous or oral injection is usually used.

Chemotherapy drugs can

- Defect or prevent cell division. This is what cytotoxic drugs do.
- Target the food source of the cell and do not allow the necessary hormones and enzymes to reach the cancer cell.
- Encourage cancer cells to commit suicide. In medical terms, this is called a storage cell.
- Preventing the formation and growth of new capillaries that are responsible for supplying blood to the cancerous gland. Of course, the effectiveness of this method has been questioned in recent years.

Chemotherapy and its relationship with stem cells

Some researchers have shown that if instead of starving a cancer cell, we prevent blood from reaching it, we may increase its resistance to treatment and increase the possibility of metastasis. On the other hand, more studies have convinced scientists that using the same methods may still be effective. Scientists have suggested that if we target proteins that are overexpressed by cancer, we can reduce the risk of resistance to treatment or the possibility of metastasis. Stem cell therapy is the use of stem cells to treat or prevent a disease or condition.

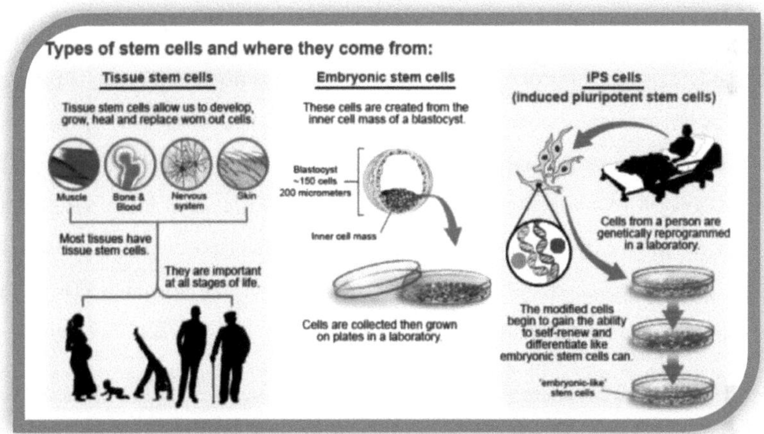

Figure 17. Stem cells and regenerative medicine

Bone marrow transplant

Bone marrow transplant is the most common stem cell treatment, but some cord blood treatments are also being used. Research is underway to develop various sources of stem cells as well as stem cell therapy for neurological diseases and conditions such as diabetes, heart disease, etc. After developments such as the ability of scientists to isolate and culture embryonic stem cells, the creation of stem cells using the transfer of the nucleus of somatic cells and their use as methods of creating pluripotent stem cells derived from stem cells has become controversial. This disagreement is often related to the politics of abortion and human cloning. In addition, marketing efforts based on stored umbilical cord blood transplantation have been controversial.

For more than 30 years, bone marrow has been used to treat cancer patients with conditions such as leukemia and lymphoma. This is the only type of cell therapy that is widely used. During chemotherapy, most of the growing cells are killed by cytotoxic agents. However, these agents cannot differentiate between leukemia or neoplastic cells and hematopoietic stem cells in the bone marrow. This is a side effect of conventional chemotherapies that the stem cell transplant attempts to reverse. Healthy donor bone marrow provides functional stem cells to replace cells lost in the host's body during treatment. The transplanted cells also trigger an immune response that helps kill the cancer cells. This process can go too far, but leads to graft-versus-host disease, the most serious side effect of this treatment. Stem cells are studied for many reasons. Also, molecules and exosomes released from stem cells are studied for the preparation of drugs. In addition to the function of the cells themselves, paracrine soluble factors produced by stem cells known as stem cell secretion are another mechanism. Treatment methods based on stem cells have their effects in degenerative diseases, immunity and inflammatory diseases mediated by the immune system.

Use of peripheral blood bank

In other words, there are different types of cells in the peripheral blood bank, including red blood cells, white blood cells, platelets, and hematopoietic precursor cells; In this bank, cancer cells divide more than healthy cells. Therefore, chemotherapy and radiation therapy are used in this method to treat cancer. Chemotherapy and radiation therapy affect the speed of cell division. Bone marrow cells are destroyed by chemotherapy and radiation therapy, and stem cells are called to restore these lost cells; Stem cells called to the peripheral blood can be a useful source for reviving the hematopoietic system and the patient's immune system after severe chemotherapy.

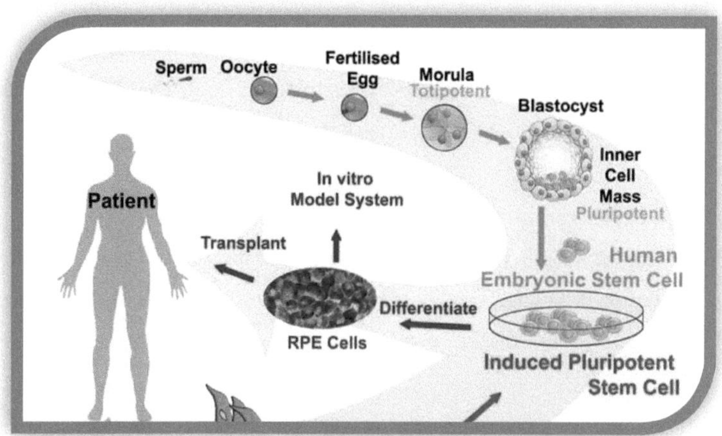

Figure 18. Induced Pluripotent Stem Cells (iPSC): Meaning, Function and Significance

Stem cell replaces chemotherapy in the repair of solid tumors. Today, autologous peripheral blood stem cell transplantation is widely used in the treatment of cancers that are treated with high-dose chemotherapy; This method is not only used for blood cancers, but also for solid tumors that are sensitive to chemotherapy, including breast cancer and small cell lung cancer. Also, some researches show that sequential injection of peripheral blood stem cells can increase the intensity and power of chemotherapy. The purpose of stem cells in the peripheral blood bank is to freeze these stem cells, which is considered a suitable treatment method for long-term storage of these cells in order to help patients.

Results of cell therapy in patients

After a short period of time, patients feel that they have increased energy and that their internal powers have improved. These patients experience favorable results in the treatment of the loss of mental pressure and improvement of mental and psychological activities. The restored functional activity of the damaged and weakened internal organs and tissues leads to a uniform recovery. Treatment with this method has led to positive results in the treatment of cancer, AIDS, diabetes, sclerosis and chronic diseases and more than 50 other diseases. Cell therapy helps prevent tumor growth and can be used to prevent disease and its recurrence.

What is disc degeneration?

One of the most common causes of back pain is disc degeneration or destruction of the internal tissue of the discs, which can be related to the discs of the back, neck or spine. The inside of the disc is made of a hard gelatin-like substance that is a collection of collagens + proteoglycan. In terms of oxygen supply, discs are considered among the tissues with low oxygen supply and due to the lack of blood vessels due to mechanical pressure, aging or inflammatory diseases, they are very vulnerable. As a result of these injuries, the internal tissue of the disc undergoes changes that reduce the flexibility of the disc and the disc slowly deteriorates. This type of damage to the disc causes chronic back pains that are associated with dryness and cramping in the area on both sides of the spine. Degenerative changes are one of the most common causes of chronic and treatment-resistant back pain in those who have back pain due to improper working conditions or aging.

From which sources can stem cells be obtained in adults?
Two important sources for obtaining stem cells are
- ➢ **Bone marrow:** The process of extracting stem cells in this way is painful, and 50,000 to 60,000 cells are extracted each time.
- ➢ **Fat:** Using very minimally invasive liposuction, about 40 million stem cells are removed from abdominal fat in a 20-minute process with local anesthesia.

Can this work be done in all patients with lumbar disc disease?

This treatment is related to discs that have been damaged and destroyed, so-called degeneration, and certain age and diagnostic criteria are necessary for the patient to be a candidate for lumbar disc cell therapy. Compliance with specialized criteria in the use of this method in disc treatment can be the reason for the success of this treatment method and it cannot be performed in all discs.

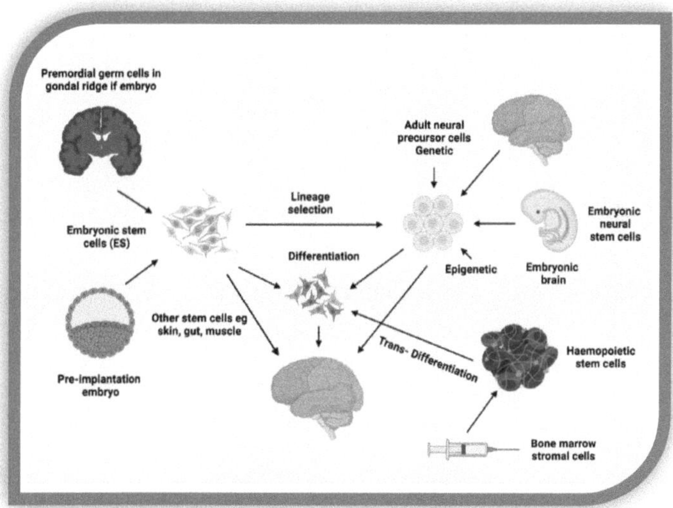

Figure 19. Stem Cell Transplantation Therapy and Neurological Disorders: Current Status and Future Perspectives

Chapter III

The effect of Stem Cell in Stomach Cancer

As you know, prevention is always better than cure. In addition to affecting people's morale, malignant stomach cancer also has significant costs. This cancer can affect the side organs, lymph nodes, pancreas, esophagus and stomach. It may even enter the liver, lungs and other organs with the blood. In other words, it spreads to the whole body with the lymphatic system. Although the causes of stomach cancer are not known 100%, doctors recommend following a few things to prevent the occurrence of cancer as much as possible. To reduce the risk of stomach cancer, it is better to observe the following things.

- ➢ Avoid drinking alcohol.
- ➢ Pay attention to fitness. If you are underweight or overweight, talk to your doctor about weight control and try to maintain a healthy weight, not so fat that you put your health at risk, and not so thin that you are weak and unable to do anything.
- ➢ Reduce consumption of red meat and its processed derivatives.
- ➢ Do not use fast foods and prepared foods as much as possible.
- ➢ Feeding babies with breast milk helps prevent cancer.
- ➢ Do not rely too much on dietary supplements.
- ➢ Give special importance to sports.
- ➢ Have a diet full of fruits and vegetables. Try to use more fruits and vegetables in your diet. Fruits and vegetables are rich in fiber and antioxidants, which greatly help to treat and prevent stomach cancer.
- ➢ Reduce salty and smoked foods. To avoid stomach cancer, keep your stomach safe from the bite of smoked and salty foods that come into contact with stomach cells directly after swallowing. Limit the use of such foods to once a month.
- ➢ Avoid using drugs and smoking. If you are addicted to smoking, especially tobacco, be sure to limit its use and stop it completely. Even if you have never gone to a tobacco shop, I recommend that you never go there and guarantee your health.

Refer to a specialist doctor

At the time of observing the symptoms, keep calm and consult your general or family doctor. Refer to a radiation oncologist after making sure you have no other gastrointestinal disease. You must know your medical history to answer the doctor's questions correctly. Talking about your history is also especially helpful. If necessary, be sure to have someone with you. Note that the first days of observing the symptoms of stomach cancer are one of the golden opportunities that should not be missed. Be sure to ask the questions you want and solve the ambiguous points. Specialists with sufficient experience and advertisement will provide the most optimal solution. Fortunately, new methods are being developed to treat stomach cancer every day.

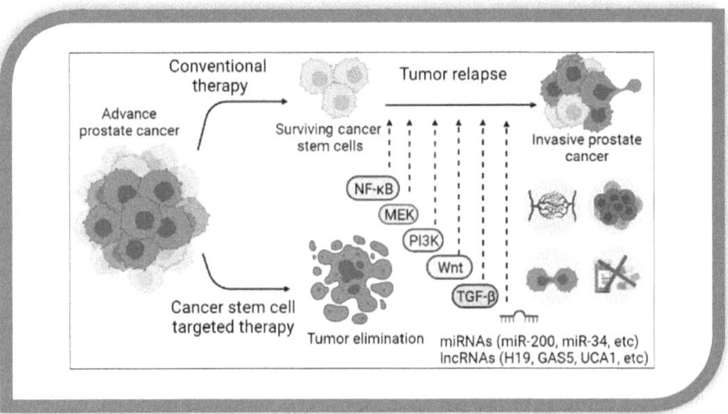

Figure 20. Signaling Pathways and Targeted Therapies for Stem Cells in Prostate Cancer

Comprehensive information about breast cancer

If we look around us, we will see that breast cancer is progressing significantly and its prevalence among women is increasing every day. All women should do annual breast screenings and see a gynecologist as soon as they notice changes in their breasts. Many of the symptoms of cancer are diagnosed by the person himself, and the earlier the diagnosis, the more successful the treatment.

What is breast cancer?

Breasts consist of a set of glands and ducts that transport milk to the nipples. But breast cancer occurs when the cells lining the glands and ducts grow uncontrollably and irregularly, and this growth continues to the extent that it spreads through the blood and lymph to all parts of the body. Breast cancer is one of the most common types of cancer in the world and its prevalence is increasing day by day.

How many types of breast cancer are there?

If breast cancer is hereditary in your family, from the age of 35 onwards, perform a mammography test (breast imaging) every year under the supervision of a gynecologist. It should be noted that breast lumps are cancerous. It takes 10 years for a fat gland to grow to one centimeter. This disease causes an increase in the deposition of ESR and an increase in kleistotin. Breast cancer is divided into two main groups:

> **INSITO group (in place)**

The reason is the deformed cells that are the origin of these cancer cells inside the mammary glands that have not invaded other parts, which is completely the primary range.

> **INVASIVE group**

Breast fibroma

They are called benign breast glands, which are common under the age of 30.

Mastectomy

It is called surgical removal of the breast.

Common breast masses are

- Lipoma;
- Fat necrosis;
- Infection; Adenoma fibroma (mostly seen in young women);
- Cystic disease.

What symptoms can breast cancer have?

If you notice the symptoms of breast cancer in time, the treatment will definitely be more effective. Cancer can start in different parts of the breast. Cancer in each part of the breast has different symptoms, for example, cancer in the milk ducts may be associated with the symptoms of a lump, and cancer in the glands may be associated with the symptoms of breast thickness. But in general, the most important early signs and symptoms of breast cancer include the following:

- Presence of mass in the breast tissue;
- Changes in the appearance of the skin or nipple.

How does cancer progress in the body?

However, the following symptoms are warning signs of breast cancer, and if you see them, you should definitely visit a doctor or a specialized clinic.

- Breast skin changes such as swelling and redness;
- Changes in the size and shape of the breasts;
- Change in the appearance of the nipples;
- Presence of pain in any part of the breast;
- Touching the lump or knot inside the breast.

In some cases, more aggressive cancer symptoms are seen, which include

➢ Breast itching or inflammation and breast discoloration;

➢ Increase the volume of the breasts in a short period of time;

➢ Sensation of changes in the breasts when touched;

➢ Scaling of the nipples;

➢ Redness or dimpling of the skin of the breasts like the peel of an orange;

➢ Swelling or lump in the lymph nodes;

➢ Nipple discharge.

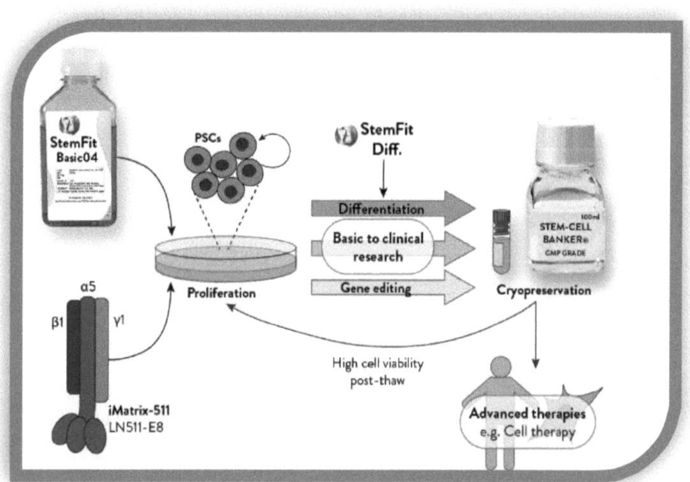

Figure 21. Stem Cell Synergy Solution

What causes breast cancer?

One of the most important causes of breast cancer is mutation or change in the DNA of breast cells. But we subcategorize the important factors that cause cancer.

General factors

Aging becomes one of the main causes of breast cancer. Usually, women over 60 years old are more susceptible to cancer, and a small percentage of women under 40 years old get breast cancer. Gender is another general factor that occurs in women a hundred times more often than in men, and about 1% of men in the world are affected by this cancer.

Genetic factors

One of the most important genetic factors involved in causing cancer is family history, usually women whose mother, sister, or daughter have been diagnosed with cancer are twice as likely to develop it. Hereditary gene mutations are also effective in the occurrence of cancer, which is the most common mutation related to BRCA1 and BRCA2 genes.

Factors related to the body system

Obesity and overweight is one of the things that plays a key role in many diseases. The breast tissue is dense. Breast changes are important. Menstrual status should be taken seriously. All these cases are involved in the occurrence of cancer.

Factors related to lifestyle

Unhealthy lifestyle that is continuously insisted on, you will suffer from various diseases such as cancer.

> - Lack of physical activity;
> - Lack of exercise and physical activity;
> - Drinking alcoholic beverages.

Stages of breast cancer expansion

Grading of the stages of breast cancer spread is different based on the type of cancer and in which part of the breast it is observed. Determining the steps helps the treatment. The stages of breast cancer are as follows:

Clinical stage

Any information obtained through primary diagnoses such as ultrasound, MRI, and mammography.

Pathological stage

Necessary tests on the removed tissue samples and their evaluation.

Note: More staging is done to determine the size of the tumor and its spread.

TNM system

The most common method for staging cancer is the TNM system. This system examines the size of the tumor, its progression and spread to the lymph nodes, and the extent of the spread of cancer in other parts of the body.

What diagnostic methods are there for breast cancer?

Unfortunately, there is no national screening for breast cancer in Iran. While in many countries of the world, including England, all women who are over 50 years old get a mammogram every three years. For this reason, the number of deaths caused by breast cancer in the UK has decreased drastically due to the early detection of breast cancer. By regularly examining their breasts, they can feel lumps in their breasts. Most of the lumps in the breast are benign. For this reason, it is better for people not to worry and check themselves every month after their monthly habits.

What should be done for the personal examination of people?

For a personal breast examination, the upper bodice should be removed first. Then he stood in front of the mirror and put his hands on his waist so that his shoulders are in a line and note that we should look for these symptoms in the personal examination of the breast.

> Bump – Changing the size and shape of the breast;

> Discharge from the nipple;

> Redness or eczema;

> Prominence of veins;

> Skin wear or wrinkles;

> Indentation of the nipple or changing of the nipple.

Note that these observations should be checked in another position, that is, the hands are on the sides and these observations and checks are done again, or that we bend forward so that the breasts hang down.

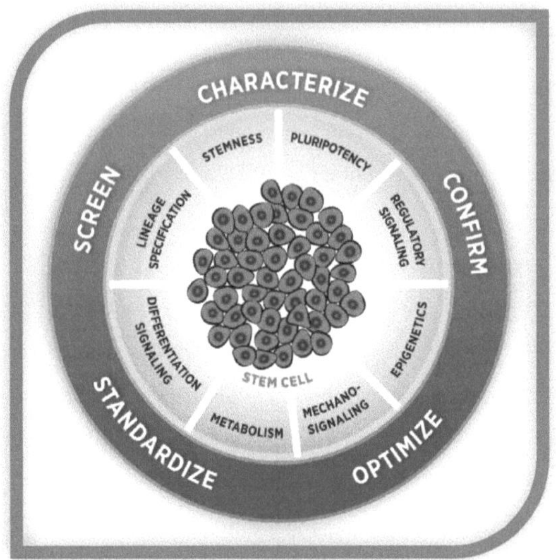

Figure 22. nCounter® Stem Cell Characterization Panel

If we find a problem, it is definitely necessary to go to the breast cancer treatment center, and if we do not find it, we must touch it. To touch it, you must stick all four fingers together, we consider the soft part of the finger and place it on your breast and we start looking for the mass with circular movements on the chest, and to be sure, it is better to press the hand more so that if you have a mass, you can touch it. Note that the most important part to find the mass is the part of the breast that extends to the armpit. The reason why we say to put the hand under the head is that the part of the breast is completely stretched so that you can find it by pressing on the face of the mass. Prevention of breast cancer can depend on doing these examinations, so don't neglect it.

Mammography

Mammography method is used to take pictures of the internal structure of breasts, which is performed by X-rays. For people who are suspected of having cancer, this method quickly detects cancer in the early stages and makes the treatment process start earlier and more effectively.

Ultrasound

This method works by sound waves. If a person's symptoms are suspicious of cancer, ultrasound is prescribed for more detailed investigations. The advantage of this method is to distinguish pseudo masses from real abnormal masses, which is known as one of the auxiliary methods for breast cancer diagnosis.

MRI

This method recognizes the nature of hidden masses by detecting them. Among the various applications of this method, there are cases such as breast examination of people who had problems in the initial diagnosis. People with breast surgery, people with previous history of breast cancer and suspected of disease recurrence, etc.

Sampling or biopsy

If suspicious lumps are observed in the breast in the previous methods, the sampling method should be used for a more definitive diagnosis.

Breast cancer in men

Breast cancer is not exclusive to women, but it is possible for men to get breast cancer as well. Because of the breast tissue that men have, it is possible for the cells to be involved in cancer cells. However, breast cancer in men is very rare and usually occurs in old age.

Symptoms of breast cancer in men

Considering that breast cancer is very common in women, the presence of this disease has also been seen in men. Considering that this cancer is rare, it should not be ignored. As a result, you should know the symptoms so that you can see a doctor quickly.

> Discharge from the breast;

> Thickening of breast tissue;

> Nipple redness;

> Skin sensitivity or itching;

> Turning the nipple inwards;

> Build mass.

According to research, it has been shown that cancer diagnosis occurs later in men because men do not check their breast tissue regularly.

Examination to diagnose breast cancer

In case of any mass or pain in the chest area, it is better to see a doctor quickly so that diagnostic procedures can be performed.

> **Physical examination:** The doctor examines the chest and skin well.

> **Medical history:** It is better to inform your doctor about any medicine you use, and if you have a family history, tell your doctor because breast cancer is one of the diseases that are related to genes.

> **Mammogram:** It is an X-ray scan that detects the mass well.

> **Ultrasound:** It is performed for the purpose of imaging the tissue and to diagnose breast cancer.

> **MRI:** Sometimes the doctor requests MRI along with other tests. It is a non-invasive method and is performed for imaging purposes.
> **Biopsy:** It is done by removing a small part of the tissue for a more detailed examination.

Note that timely diagnosis of cancer is very sensitive and important because the sooner breast cancer is diagnosed, the easier it is to recover. Therefore, if you are suffering from breast cancer or have doubts about it, you can go to the best breast cancer treatment center or the best cancer treatment center to treat this cancer.

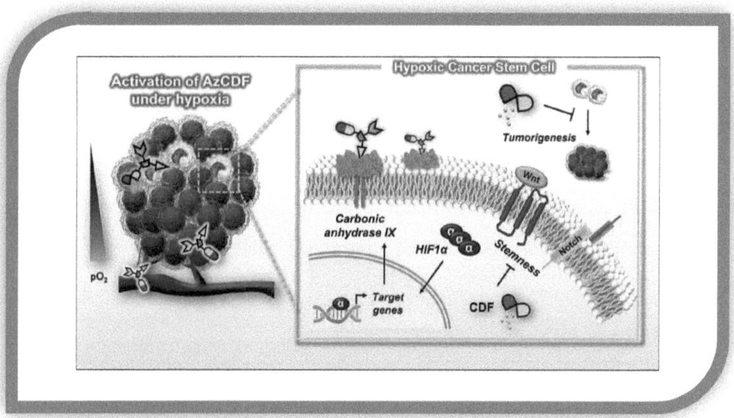

Figure 23. A Small Molecule Strategy for Targeting Cancer Stem Cells in Hypoxic Microenvironments and Preventing Tumorigenesis

Laryngeal cancer, cause, treatment and diagnosis of larynx cancer

Unfortunately, recently, cancer has become widespread. This disease is one of the dangerous diseases that threaten human life. Laryngeal cancer occurs due to a change in the covering of the larynx, which is caused by long-term irritation of the larynx (usually with cigarette smoke, etc.). Cancer of the larynx or throat is a dangerous disease that affects the vocal cords and larynx or a part of the throat and causes swallowing problems and disturbances in speech and may also damage the lymph nodes in the head and neck. The advanced type that involves the lymph nodes is very dangerous and endangers human life.

1.284.3 Causes of laryngeal cancer

There are many reasons that increase the risk of developing laryngeal cancer, including

- ➢ Consumption of all kinds of tobacco, including cigarettes and hookah, etc.
- ➢ Excessive drinking of alcoholic beverages. People who drink too much alcohol are more prone to this disease.
- ➢ People who are exposed to mustard gas and dangerous radiation.
- ➢ People who deal with wood chips a lot.
- ➢ Severe and strong gastric reflux can cause this disease.

It should be noted that the appearance of one or more of the above symptoms is not necessarily the cause of laryngeal cancer, but it can be said that a person who has the above symptoms is more at risk of contracting this disease.

1.284.4 Symptoms of laryngeal cancer

Laryngeal cancer can have many symptoms; we mention some of them

- ➢ Feeling of shortness of breath and swallowing disorders;
- ➢ Significant change in voice, usually the voice becomes softer and these changes are noticeable by friends, acquaintances and people who are always in contact with the patient;
- ➢ Severe pain in the ear area;
- ➢ Sputum or blood coming out when coughing;
- ➢ Chronic cough that never gets better;
- ➢ Feeling long-term pain in the throat area (this pain lasts for at least six consecutive weeks).

Laryngeal cancer is a common type that will be much easier to treat if it is diagnosed early and timely treatment can cause a complete recovery of this disease. Usually, this cancer occurs in people over 60 years' old who have been smoking for a long time.

What is ovarian cancer? Symptoms and treatment of ovarian cancer

Ovarian cancer is a silent killer?! Ovarian cancer has been called the "Silent killer" because its symptoms usually appear when the disease has reached advanced stages and is mostly incurable. But health experts have identified a set of physical symptoms that occur in women with ovarian cancer and may be early warning signs for this disease. These symptoms are very common and most of the women who show them do not have ovarian cancer. But for women with ovarian cancer, the hope is that more awareness about them will lead to early diagnosis and treatment of the disease.

The American Cancer Society and the American Society of Gynecologic Oncologists emphasize these four symptoms as symptoms that are more common in women with ovarian cancer than in the general population: Burping and increasing the size of the abdomen; Abdominal or pelvic pain; Difficulties in eating and early satiety and frequency and urgency of urination. According to this guideline, any woman who experiences one or more of these symptoms almost every day for several weeks should see a clinical doctor, preferably a gynecologist, to undergo a pelvic examination. If a person's pelvic examination is suspicious, it is usually followed by a non-invasive diagnostic method, vaginal ultrasound and possibly blood measurement of a cancer indicator called CA-125. The only way to definitively diagnose ovarian cancer is during surgery, which is best done by a gynecologist who has experience in the field of ovarian cancer.

Research has shown that many women with ovarian cancer have complained of the symptoms mentioned above long before the diagnosis of cancer, but these symptoms were either ignored or attributed to other diseases. The four symptoms that were mentioned occur in many other diseases such as menstrual disorders, irritable bowel syndrome and bladder infections. But if such symptoms occur without previous history, continue for several weeks and worsen over time, they may be a sign of ovarian cancer.

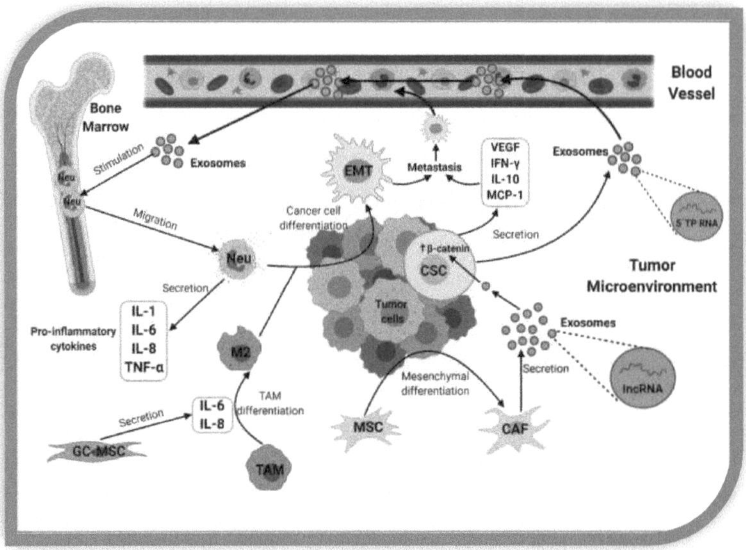

Figure 24. The cross talk between gastric cancer stem cells and the immune microenvironment: a tumor-promoting factor, Stem Cell Research & Therapy

Ovarian cancer in women

Ovarian cancer is a silent killer for women. This fatal disease is related to the reproductive system of women and according to the obtained statistics, it kills 15,000 women every year. The reason is that 80% of the time this disease is discovered when it is too late, that is, when the cancer has spread to other organs. But fortunately, doctors discover the basic secrets of this disease and these discoveries can save your life.

Diagnosis of ovarian cancer

There are three general stages to diagnose ovarian cancer. A general examination that includes a pelvic examination. Ultrasound is one of the diagnostic methods for ovarian cancer. A blood test is necessary for an accurate diagnosis.

Why should we pay attention to the warning signs of ovarian cancer?

The ovaries release hormones (estrogen and progesterone) and because of this, the eggs are released from the follicle, but deep inside the ovary, healthy cells become cancerous and gradually attack the rest of the tissues and gradually grow larger. And they enter the uterine tubes and enter other parts of the body, and it becomes difficult to diagnose cancer. Because they are surrounded by other organs of the body and here the work of doctors becomes difficult and they cannot diagnose well. If dear patients pay attention to the symptoms of cancer, they can be treated well.

Symptoms of ovarian cancer

Usually, the age of onset of this cancer is between 50 and 60 years old, and if the person is diagnosed earlier than this age, the diagnosis becomes a little more difficult. When ovarian cancer is diagnosed in the early stages, 90% of the treatment is done, but when it is treated late, the chance of treatment is between 20 and 30%.

- Abdominal enlargement;
- Flatulence;
- Stomach ache;
- Intestinal pain;
- Pelvic pain;
- Difficulty in eating and feeling full too soon.

If you feel such symptoms every day or every other day for several weeks, it is necessary to see a doctor and it is better to know that it is not necessary to have all the symptoms to diagnose cancer. If you have only one of these symptoms and it continues for several weeks, you should see a doctor.

Kidney cancer with ways to recognize types of kidney cancer

Is kidney cancer fatal? What is the treatment of kidney cancer? About 3% of all adult malignancies are uncommon, and the ratio of men to women is 3:2, which increases with age, and 75% occur in men over 60 years old.

Causes of kidney cancer

Kidney cancer is often asymptomatic; it is a random finding in screening tests. The classic three symptoms of hematuria, flank pain and abdominal mass are only in 10% of patients.

- Smoking;
- Obesity;
- Tuberous sclerosis;
- Acquired polycystic kidney disease (chronic dialysis).

Symptoms of kidney cancer malignancy

If a person experiences weight loss, fatigue, paraneoplastic syndromes, fever of unknown origin, and symptoms of hypercalcemia or polycythemia, it means that the person has malignant symptoms and should see a doctor immediately.

Examination of kidney cancer

There may be no symptoms. Increased blood pressure, local anemia or hyperemia, palpable renal mass, left tumor may spread to the left renal vein, which can lead to left testicular vein obstruction and left varicocele. Leads. In one third of the cases, there is a metastasis.

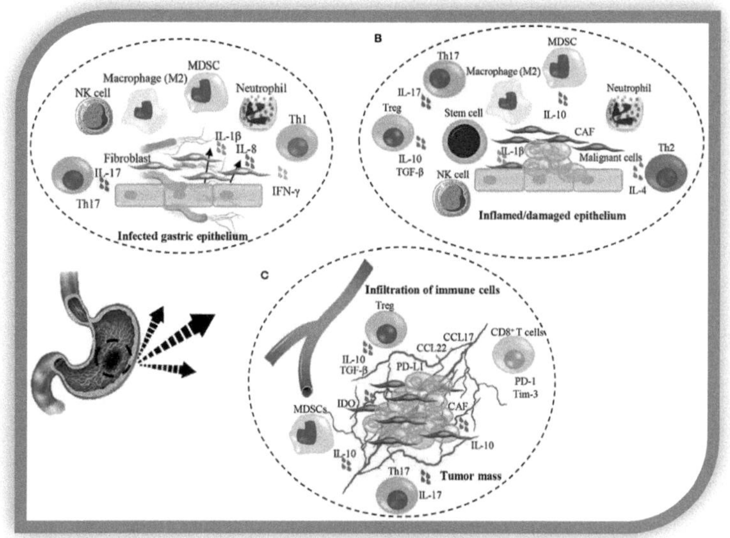

Figure 25. Gastric Cancer Stem Cells Effect on Th17/Treg Balance; A Bench to Beside Perspective

Diagnosis of kidney cancer

> **Urine:** Using a test strip (to detect hematuria), urine cytology.

> **Blood:** Complete blood cell count, urea and electrolytes, calcium, liver function tests.

> **Imaging:** Ultrasound, CT scan or MRI, PET or bone scan to check for metastasis.

> **Abdominal ultrasound:** The most useful examination is the first line of diagnostic procedures. With it, solid masses can be distinguished from cystic types. The use of KUB and IVU is limited, and with these methods, only large lesions that change the borders of the kidney or the ureter They are diagnosed with pressure, CT scan with contrast and MRI are more sensitive and make staging possible.

- ➢ **Pathology:** Histological types include types of clear cells, chromophilic, chromophobic, oncocytoma and collecting duct tumor.
- ➢ **Robson staging:** Stage 1 tumor inside the kidney capsule, 2 spread to the fat around the kidney but not niam grota, stage 3 invasion of the renal veins, inferior vena cava or regional lymph nodes, stage 4 spread to nearby viscera or distant metastasis.

Kidney cancer along with treatment

Surgery for the treatment of kidney cancer includes radical nephrectomy, along with the removal of fat around the kidney, grotta's fascia, adrenal gland on the side of the lesion, and regional enphadenectomy is the standard treatment. It may be done by peritoneal, lateral, thoracoabdominal or laparoscopic approach.

Radiotherapy and chemotherapy: Renal cell cancer is highly resistant to chemotherapy drugs (which is due to glycoprotein G resistant to several drugs). A good response is possible with the use of new T-kinase inhibitors such as sorafenib and sonitinib. Radiotherapy may be used in lesions with metastasis.

Complications of kidney cancer

Distant metastasis (50% of lung cases and 33% of bone cases). Local invasion (including obstruction of the inferior vena cava and invasion of the fat around the kidney), local bleeding, colic caused by a clot, paraneoplastic syndromes.

Prognosis of kidney cancer

It depends on the type and stage of the tumor. With stage 1 tumor removal, the 5-year survival rate is 94% in cases of lymph node invasion 18-30% and with distant metastasis 0-20%. Testicular cancer, testicular cancer diagnosis and prevention symptoms. Testicular cancer is a type of cancer that usually affects one testicle. This disease is one of the most common diseases in men. This type may occur at any age, even between the ages of 15 and 38. The probability of treating this disease will be higher if it is diagnosed early. In the following, we intend to talk about this type of disease and its prevention, diagnosis and treatment methods in general.

What is testicular cancer?

Testicles are male sexual organs that are responsible for sperm production and storage. These two organs are placed in a bag called scrotum under the penis. As mentioned, testicular cancer is one of the most common types of cancer that occurs when abnormal cells grow uncontrollably in the testicle. If the development of this type of cells is not significant, this disease can be treated.

What are the symptoms of testicular cancer?

It usually involves one testicle. If you observe any swelling, pain and the following symptoms, if it lasts more than two weeks, see a specialist doctor.

- Finding a hard lump in one or both testicles;
- Enlargement of the testicles;
- Feeling of heaviness in the scrotum (the bag that covers the testicles.);
- Pain and discomfort in the lower abdomen or genitals;
- Condensation of fluids in the scrotum;
- Increasing or decreasing the size of the testicles;
- Pain in the chest and breasts in men;
- Pain and discomfort in the scrotum;
- Increase in volume and any changes in male breast.

What are the causes of testicular cancer?

The causes of testicular cancer are still unknown, but there are factors that increase the risk of developing this disease, which include:

Intra-abdominal testis

The meaning of intra-abdominal testicle is that the testicle stays inside the abdomen and is not placed in the scrotum, which is used to remove it during surgery. Among the complications of intra-abdominal testicles, sperm weakness and infertility can also be mentioned.

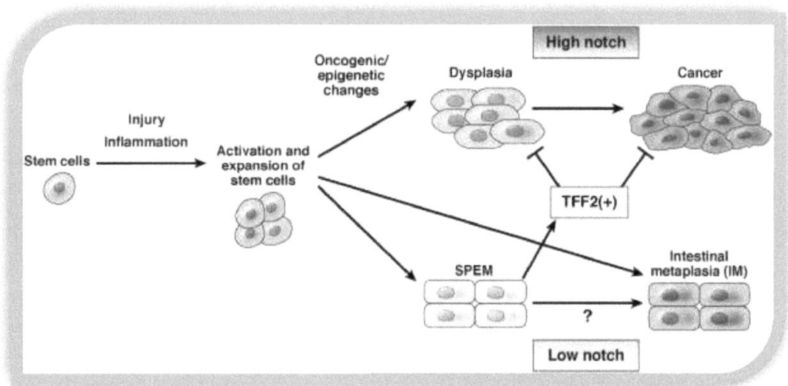

Figure 26. The Origins of Gastric Cancer From Gastric Stem Cells: Lessons From Mouse Models

Testicular cancer

It may happen at any age, but it is obvious that the risk of developing testicular cancer increases with age.

Hereditary and genetic factors

It can also be effective in getting testicular cancer. If there is an infected person in the family, the risk will increase.

What methods are there to diagnose testicular cancer?

If you feel any lump in your testicles, see a doctor immediately. If there is a possibility of testicular cancer, you should go to the hospital for additional tests and sampling (biopsy). If cancer is diagnosed, the testicle and the lymph tissues around it are completely removed, and chemotherapy and radiation therapy are used to prevent the recurrence of the disease. The mentioned measures are conditional on the diagnosis of cancer in the early stages. It is recommended to examine the testicles by the person himself. The most suitable time for examination is when the scrotum is relaxed. Gently squeeze the testicle between your fingers. If there is any hard mass, see a doctor immediately.

How can testicular cancer be prevented?

Do you know what factors increase the risk of testicular cancer? When cancer cells start to act in one or both testes and form a mass or tumor. These cancer cells can also transfer to the bloodstream and spread throughout the body, which is another name for metastasis. Many men who have this type of cancer, no scientific reason has been proven for it. But some of the known reasons for this type of cancer are hidden testicles (the testicles are formed in the baby's abdomen and after birth are transferred to the shell outside the abdomen, but in rare cases, the testicles remain in the abdomen), white skin and family history that cannot be prevented. Accordingly, prevention is not possible in many cases. However, identifying testicular cancer in the early stages helps the treatment process. Here are some signs that you should pay attention to:

- Feeling a gland or excessive size of one of the testicles;
- Feeling of heaviness in the testicles;
- Mild pain in the lower abdomen or groin;
- Sudden collection of a large amount of fluid in the scrotum;
- Pain or discomfort in the scrotum;
- Breast size or tenderness;
- Pain in the back and lower back.

What are the treatment methods for malignant testicular cancer?

For the treatment of cancers, we face a main question whether it can be treated or not. This type of cancer can be treated ninety-nine percent of the time, and even in the case of testicular cancer metastasis, it can be treated in most cases. The treatment of malignant type is combined with chemotherapy and surgery. First of all, the type of testicular cancer must be diagnosed for treatment, which in most cases, the doctor diagnoses it as seminoma and non-seminoma by examining the patient and checking his age. Ninety-five percent of patients between 25 and 45 years of age suffer from testicular cancer of the simnomia type. When the tumor is 5 cm or less, the tumor is surgically removed. After that radiation therapy of lymph nodes and pelvis is necessary to complete the treatment course. Most tumors are a combination of seminoma and non-seminoma cancer cells, and this issue does not overshadow the treatment method.

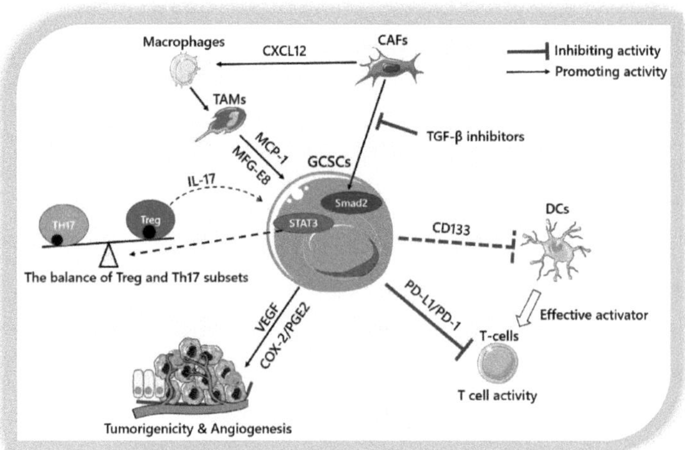

Figure 27. Gastric Cancer Stem Cells: Current Insights into the Immune Microenvironment and Therapeutic Targets

Leukemia symptoms and the best leukemia treatment center

Leukemia, despite medical advances, cancer is still one of the most terrible diagnoses that a patient can receive from his doctor. Regarding this disease, do you think there is a cure for leukemia? Blood cancers are one of the most common types of cancer that affect blood cells and bone marrow - the spongy tissue inside your bones where blood cells are made. These cancers change the way blood cells behave and function. Blood cells have major functions in the body, which include

- White blood cells fight infection as part of the body's immune system.
- Red blood cells carry oxygen to body tissues and organs and carry carbon dioxide to your lungs so you can breathe it.
- Platelets can help blood clot after wound formation.

Silent cancer called leukemia

When we live in a world where getting cancer is as common as a simple cold, it is natural that when we see a small sign, our mind goes towards cancer. It is as if we are living in a world of diseases, and instead of building a healthy life, we should look for a way to build a disease-free life. Living with cancer is more like fighting than living. If we change our perspective a little, we can also conclude that if there were no outbreaks of diseases, medical science would not have progressed and mankind would have been satisfied with the same basic sciences of the past centuries. Although a large number of people have become victims of this development, they have been able to improve the quality of life of the next generations and turn the early humans into the current humans with this amount of awareness. Therefore, cancer or any other severe disease has two aspects, which are bitter and sweet.

What is leukemia?

Blood cancer starts from the stem cells in the brain and bones. A stem cell remains like a baby to some extent, that is, something that has not yet grown but has many capabilities. Many stem cells find specialized functions and become cells of organs such as liver, brain and heart. But in some tissues, they can divide into new stem cells throughout the adult growth period to continuously produce new cells and keep up with the needs of the body. For example, brain and bone, where stem cells are derived into different types of blood cells, including red cells that deliver oxygen from the lungs to other tissues, platelets that prevent bleeding by sticking to damaged vessels, and white blood cells. They protect the body and destroy dangerous invaders. Sometimes, during the specialization process of stem cells, an error occurs and dangerous mutations occur in the cell's DNA.

Leukemia is a type of cancer that does not show any unique symptoms in the beginning and is called a silent disease. Fortunately, this disease is known more with the help of molecular biology, and for this reason, it is a strong point for people who believe that this cancer has no cure. Leukemia, like other cancers, is caused by the irregular growth and proliferation of cells that float in the blood, bone marrow and lymphatic system. These cells grow in the bone marrow and disrupt the function of blood cells.

Damaged cells and DNA that are obliged to destroy themselves, but some damaged cells disobey this command and multiply uncontrollably, even while losing their main function. These are what we call cancer cells. It is not yet clear why leukemia is most common in children, but one contributing factor could be that the disease often occurs with only one or two changes in DNA. While most cancers require more changes, this makes leukemia grow faster than other cancers. In addition, some changes in DNA can happen in the embryonic stage in white blood cells and increase the risk of contracting it at a young age. Although this disease affects children more than any other cancer, the majority of those affected are adults.

When leukemia occurs, the damaged cells multiply in the brain and bones until they occupy all the available space and resources. When the bone marrow can no longer produce the required number of useful cells, the blood is depleted and reduced. The reduction of red blood cells means that the muscles cannot get enough oxygen. The low number of platelets is not enough to heal wounds, and the death of white blood cells puts the body's defense system in motion and increases the risk of infection. To restore normal blood function, cancer cells must be destroyed, but since leukemia cells do not form tumors, it is not possible to do them with surgery, instead, these cells are destroyed using different treatments.

Types of blood cancer

The three main types of blood and bone marrow cancer are: leukemia, lymphoma and myeloma

- Leukemia is a blood cancer that originates from the blood and bone marrow. It happens when the body produces too many abnormal white blood cells and interferes with the bone marrow's ability to make red blood cells and platelets.

- Non-Hodgkin's lymphoma is another type that develops in the lymphatic system from cells called lymphocytes, a type of white blood cell that helps the body fight infections.

- Hodgkin's lymphoma is a blood cancer that develops in the lymphatic system from cells called lymphocytes. Hodgkin's lymphoma is characterized by the presence of an abnormal lymphocyte called a Reed-Sternberg cell.

- Multiple myeloma is a blood cancer that starts in blood plasma cells, a type of white blood cell made in the bone marrow.

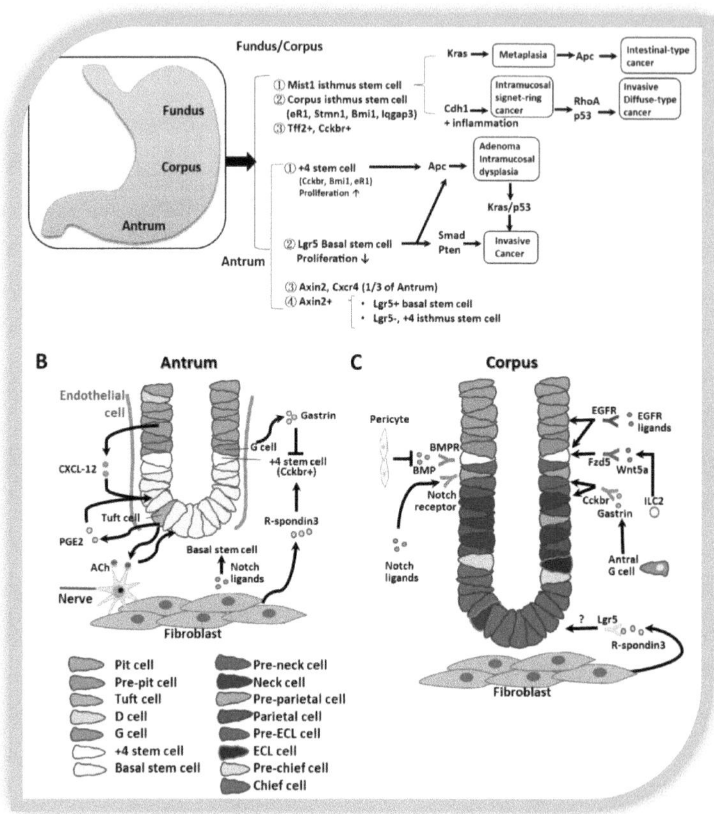

Figure 28. Generation of Human Stomach Cancer iPSC-Derived Organoids Induced by Helicobacter pylori Infection and Their Application to Gastric Cancer Research

Other types of leukemia that are less common

- ➤ **Myelodysplastic syndromes:** These are very rare diseases that occur as a result of damage to hematopoietic cells in the bone marrow.
- ➤ **Myeloproliferative neoplasms:** This type of rare blood cancer occurs when the body overproduces white blood cells, red blood cells, or platelets. Its three main branches are essential thrombocythemia, myelofibrosis and polycythemia vera.
- ➤ **Waldenström's macroglobulinemia:** This is a rare type of non-Hodgkin's lymphoma that starts from B lymphocyte cells.
- ➤ **Aplastic anemia:** This rare condition occurs when key stem cells are damaged and can only be treated with a bone marrow transplant.

Symptoms of leukemia

Extreme fatigue: This symptom is one of the main symptoms of leukemia that worsens over time.

Shortness of breath: If a person is suffering from blood cancer, he may experience shortness of breath in addition to fatigue and weakness. These people experience shortness of breath during short walks or climbing stairs. Shortness of breath is a symptom that is also observed in lung cancer and is one of the common symptoms of both. It is important that shortness of breath is caused by anemia or by the presence of a mass in the chest.

Swollen gums: One of the common symptoms of leukemia is swollen gums. Therefore, by seeing this symptom, you can know that you are suffering from this disease.

Abnormal bleeding: Abnormal bleeding is one of the signs of acute blood cancer, which is caused by a lack of platelets in the blood.

The feeling of being full or full: With the enlargement of the spleen in acute blood cancer, the appetite of patients decreases and they feel full.

Pain in the upper part of the left abdomen: This symptom, like the previous symptom, is caused by the enlargement of the spleen, because the spleen is in this part of the body, and its enlargement will cause severe pain.

Some of the common symptoms that can indicate infection are
- Ague;
- Constant fatigue;
- Weakness;
- Excessive and unreasonable weight loss;
- Abdominal discomfort;
- Headache;
- Shortness of breath.

Unusual symptoms of leukemia

Uncommon symptoms such as: Paleness, bone pain, throbbing headache, night sweats, skin rashes, swelling of the lymph nodes in the neck or armpit or groin, fever and chills, and successive infections in a specific time frame, these symptoms are generally not the main symptoms. However, it can be a suspicious symptom of this cancer.

What is the cause of leukemia?

All blood cancers are caused by mutations in the genetic material - DNA - of blood cells. Other risk factors vary based on the specific type of blood cancer.

Risk factors for acute myeloid leukemia, the most common form of leukemia in adults, are
- Increasing age;
- Gender: Which involves mostly men;

➢ Exposure to industrial chemicals such as benzene;

➢ Smoking;

➢ History of cancer treatment;

➢ Being exposed to high doses of radiation;

➢ History of other types of blood cancers.

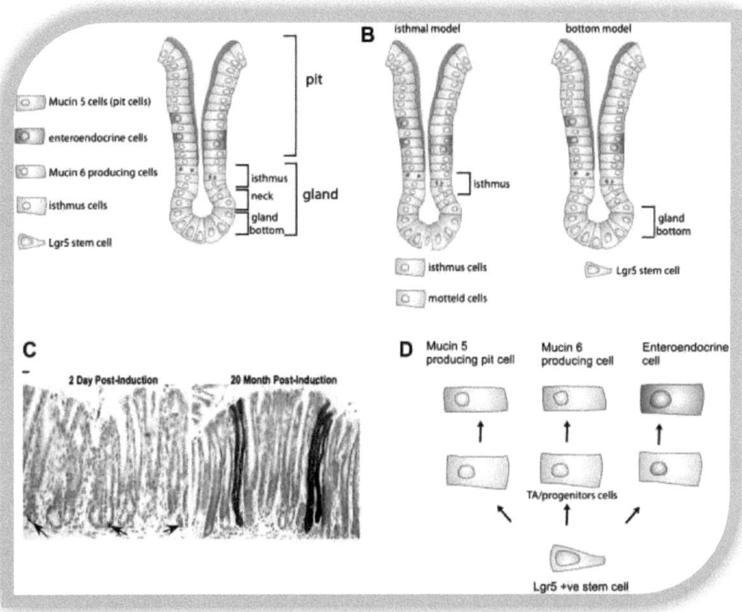

Figure 29. Stem cells and cancer of the stomach and intestine

Risk factors for developing Hodgkin's lymphoma include

➢ History of infection with Epstein-Barr virus, which causes infectious mononucleosis;

➢ Increasing age;

➢ This type of blood cancer is more common in men;

➢ Family history of Hodgkin lymphoma;

➢ Weak immune system.

Risk factors for developing non-Hodgkin's lymphoma include

➤ Being exposed to some industrial chemicals such as herbicides and insecticides;

➤ A history of chemotherapy;

➤ Exposure to radiation;

➤ Strengthening the body's immune system;

➤ History of autoimmune diseases such as rheumatoid arthritis or lupus.

Risk factors for multiple myeloma include

➤ Increasing age;

➤ Race: Higher risk among African-Americans;

➤ Obesity or overweight.

How is blood cancer diagnosed?

Making a diagnosis often begins with a physical exam to check your general health. The doctor will review your health history, examine your body and lymph nodes, and check for any signs of infection or bruising. A variety of tests and procedures may be used to diagnose leukemia. What you need depends on the type of leukemia you suspect. Your care team may recommend testing and evaluating all results with you to make a diagnosis.

Biopsy

Biopsy or sampling of cancerous tissue is a test that collects samples of cells for examination by a pathologist in the laboratory. For some types of blood cancer, such as lymphoma, you may need a lymph node biopsy, which takes a sample of lymph tissue or all lymph nodes. Blood cancer can be detected by performing a bone marrow test and sampling it. Doctors use a method called bone marrow aspiration to remove a small sample of bone marrow from the hip bone or breast bone. The smeared sample is sent to a laboratory and examined for abnormal cells or changes in genetic material.

Imaging

Imaging scans are more helpful for some types of blood cancer than others. During imaging, an enlarged lymph node may be shown, which is a common symptom of lymphoma, but it is not usually used to diagnose leukemia, a blood cancer that does not cause visible tumors. Imaging can also help determine how much blood cancer has spread in the body. Imaging required in the diagnosis of blood cancer are

> - Computed tomography (CT scan);
> - Magnetic resonance imaging (MRI);
> - Positron emission tomography scan (PET scan);
> - X-Ray;
> - Sonography.

Certain types of scans are used during a biopsy to help determine the exact area to be sampled according to the doctor's opinion.

Blood test

Complete blood cell count shows the number of cells of different blood components such as white blood cells, red blood cells and platelets. Blood chemistry tests measure the levels of important substances in your blood. For example, abnormal levels of certain proteins may provide information about your condition. If multiple myeloma is suspected, doctors may want to check your blood calcium levels. For possible lymphoma, an enzyme called lactate dehydrogenase can also be measured.

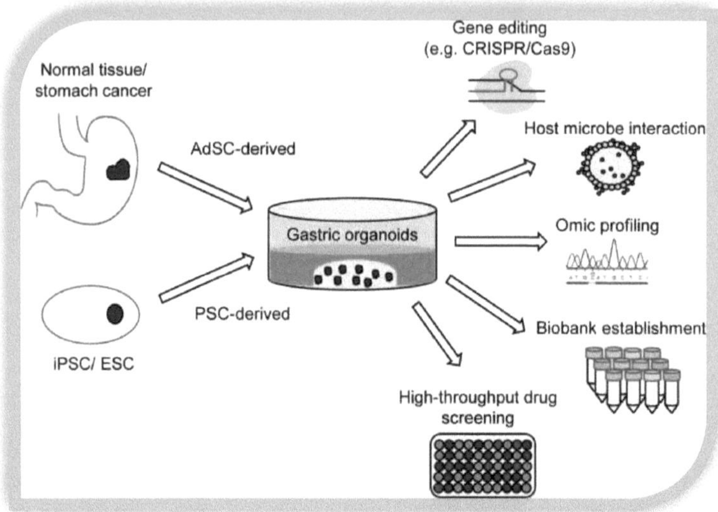

Figure 30. Stem cells and cancer of the stomach and intestine - Vries - 2010 - Molecular Oncology

Leukemia treatment

One of the methods of treating leukemia is chemotherapy, which is a combination of drugs that quickly destroy the growing cells. Unfortunately, this method also has a side effect that causes the destruction of healthy cells, such as the cells in hair follicles and intestines. Also, in some cases, the required amount of medicine is so high that it causes the death of all cells in the brain and bone, including stem cells. When this happens, the body is no longer able to produce new blood cells by itself. Fortunately, external help can be effective, mostly stem cells from the marrow and bone of a donor. After they are transplanted into the patient's body, they quickly start settling in the brain, bones, and blood. However, bone marrow transplantation is a complex process and requires antigen compatibility between the donor and the recipient to protect the transplanted cells from the attack of the patient's own cells as foreign cells. The more potential donors there are, the more patients can be saved through various transplants. So, with the increase in the number of donors, blood cancer will not look so scary anymore.

In general, blood cancer treatment is done in the following ways.

- ➢ Radiotherapy;
- ➢ Chemotherapy;
- ➢ Marrow and bone transplant and stem cell transplant in this type of blood cancer treatment, the surgeon replaces the patient's brain and bone with a healthy person so that the patient can perform chemotherapy and radiotherapy treatments well.

The type of treatment you receive for leukemia depends on several important factors, including

- ➢ Age of the patient;
- ➢ Rate of diffusion to other parts of the body;
- ➢ Medical allergy;
- ➢ History of blood cancer;
- ➢ The number of areas involved in the disease.

Common treatments for leukemia in relation to leukemia, lymphoma and multiple myeloma are

Stem cell transplant: By performing a transplant, healthy blood-forming stem cells are injected into the body. Stem cells may be collected from bone marrow, circulating blood, and umbilical cord blood and then injected into the patient's body.

Chemotherapy: Chemotherapy uses anti-cancer drugs to interfere and stop the growth of cancer cells in the body. Chemotherapy for leukemia sometimes involves the use of several drugs together in a given regimen. This treatment may also be done before stem cell transplantation.

Radiation therapy: Radiation therapy may be used to kill cancer cells or to relieve pain or discomfort. Radiation therapy is usually performed before stem cell transplantation.

Is leukemia curable?

The good news is that the cure rate for leukemia is very high. Using the right treatment and medicine can guarantee that more than half of the patients can be completely cured. The research that has been done over the years has been able to increase the survival rate of patients and the percentage of their treatment. According to the reports made at the National Institute of Health, about two-thirds of people who are diagnosed with leukemia have the possibility of living for five years or more. The cure rate for Hodgkin's and non-Hodgkin's lymphoma is 85% and 70%, respectively.

The fact is that the probability of treating leukemia is very high if it is diagnosed early and correctly, but this depends entirely on the type of cancer of the patient, his age and the stage of his disease, which shows how aggressively it has spread. The ability to treat is different according to these factors. There are blood cancers such as myeloma or chronic lymphocytic leukemia that can be effectively controlled so that the patient can live a normal and productive life for years. Always when a person is diagnosed with leukemia, the first thing you think about is whether he will recover. Yes, now, with the progress of science and the discovery and production of more effective drugs, this disease has become very treatable, but this issue is more complicated and different in children due to their young age. With the availability of targeted oral medications, chronic myelogenous leukemia is now treated like other chronic diseases such as diabetes and high blood pressure. Acute lymphoblastic leukemia, which mostly affects children, has a very high treatment capability in them, but for acute lymphoblastic leukemia and adult acute lymphoblastic leukemia, we need to take more measures to treat it in the best way.

Nutrition during leukemia

Nutrition plays an important role in supplying energy to the body and treating leukemia. You need to provide the necessary energy for your treatment during your illness and until you recover completely. In this section, we will introduce a number of important food items to you in this section:

> ➢ Improve your diet by eating more vegetables, fruits, whole grains and legumes. Eating more plants means that 25 percent or less of your meals should include animal protein, such as meat, poultry, eggs, fish, and dairy products. To get enough protein, replace animal proteins with lentils, dried beans, seeds, nuts, tofu and other plant proteins.

> ➢ Choose real foods to provide nutrients and energy. Avoid artificial supplements and foods. Real foods have more than one nutrient in them. For example, a delicious piece of fruit has fiber, multiple vitamins, carbohydrates, and water, all of which work together to fight cancer cells and regenerate healthy cells. When it comes to dietary and herbal products, natural does not mean safe.

> ➢ On the days when you have a better appetite and sense of taste, use different and more diverse foods. A change in taste is a common side effect of cancer treatment, but trying new flavors may help you manage this side effect. A new study found that leukemia patients receiving chemotherapy often prefer foods that taste sweet, slightly sweet, sour and salty rather than bitter. Patients who received meals with these flavors had a healthier weight after 30 days than patients who did not receive these flavors.

> ➢ Drink more water, tea and coffee without sweets during meals. This way, you can taste more flavors and fill up on lean protein, vegetables, grains, fruits, and healthy plant fats. Studies on tea and coffee show that both are safe to consume unless your health care team advises against them.

> ➢ Note: Green tea and green tea supplements are often recommended online and in social media posts for all cancer sufferers. Evidence that green tea prevents cancer or reduces the risk of cancer is inconclusive. Talk to your

health care team about green tea before taking any supplements or increasing your green tea intake.

> Eat foods that are safe. Food safety is important during and after cancer treatment. Cancer treatment weakens the immune system and makes the body susceptible to foodborne diseases. Read our food safety guidelines for ways to protect yourself from foodborne illness. These guidelines include information on how to prepare and store food safely and what foods to avoid.

> Note: If you have a stem cell transplant, your diet may be stricter than patients who have chemotherapy or radiation and do not have a transplant. Dietary guidelines for immunosuppressed patients vary among cancer centers. Be sure to consult your doctor about your diet.

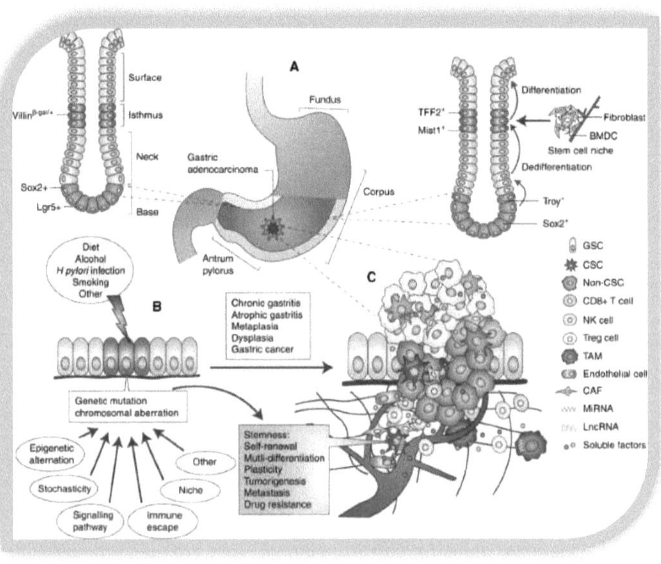

Figure 31. A unified model of the hierarchical and stochastic theories of gastric cancer

Chapter IV

Generalities of Cancer

The word neoplasm is derived from the Greek word's naos meaning new and plasis meaning formation. Therefore, neoplasm is an abnormal mass of tissue that is not useful or harmful and can also be harmful. Neoplasms are malignant or benign. The membranes of cancer cells (malignant neoplasms) are altered, thus affecting fluid transport inside and outside the cell. They also contain proteins called tumor antigens (such as PSA in prostate cancer) that make malignant cells benign. Malignant cells grow rapidly and rarely may regress spontaneously, while benign cells grow slowly and may be associated with relative periods of improvement or reduction in symptoms.

Malignant cells grow by penetrating into adjacent tissues, but benign cells grow in size and volume. Malignant cells never enter the cell, which makes it invasive to surrounding tissues and difficult to remove surgically. While benign cells are almost always inside the capsule.

The nucleus of malignant cells is large and has an abnormal shape. These cells have no physiological function and are usually anaplastic and most of its divisions are mitotic and in rare cases, if they originate from glandular tissue, they can secrete hormones.

However, benign cells rarely divide by mitosis, are not plastic, and can secrete hormones (if they originate from glandular tissue). Unlike benign cells, recurrence of malignant cells is very common. Benign cells never metastasize, while metastases (via blood and especially lymph) are very common in malignant cells. Unlike benign cells, malignant cells have certain destructive enzymes (proteinases) such as collagenase, plasminogen activator, and lysosome hydrolyzer. It destroys the host body and facilitates the invasion of the surrounding tissue. Also, these cells have less adhesion due to the small amount of fibronectin, so they can easily adhere to the surrounding structures from the original site. Malignant cells can cause wounds, infection, perforation, bleeding and dead tissue. These cells are almost always They lead to cachexia, which predisposes a person to pneumonia, anemia and other diseases.

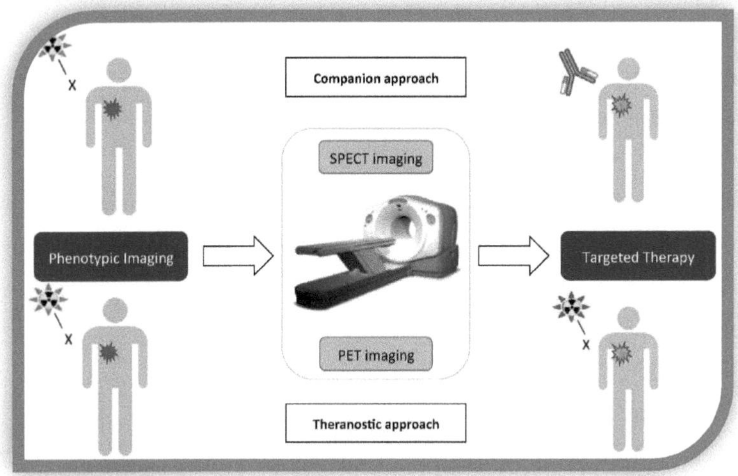

Figure 32. Cancers

Etiology

The most important causes of cancer are: physical factors, chemicals, viruses and bacteria, genetic factors, age, hormones, nutrition and the immune system.

Physical factors: Sunlight is the main source of ultraviolet radiation, which is highly carcinogenic. Bright skin, how to dress, use of canopies, humidity, altitude and latitude are effective in the amount of contact and the effect of this radiation on the body. All secondary cancers are caused by radiotherapy (especially cancer of the lung, bone, multiple myeloma, breast). Chronic irritation or inflammation also increases the risk of cancer.

Chemical agents: Cigarettes account for 30% of cancer deaths. In addition to having a direct effect on cancer, smoking exacerbates the effects of other carcinogens such as alcohol, asbestos, uranium and viruses.

2-8% of cancers are caused by contact with substances that people deal with in the workplace. Harmful substances include aromatic amines, aniline dyes, pesticides, arsenic, soot and tar, asbestos. Benzene, cadmium and chromium compounds. These substances exert their effect by altering the structure of DNA.

Liver, lungs, kidneys are at higher risk for cancer due to their special role in detoxifying chemicals from the body.

Viruses and bacteria: Viruses cause cancer by participating in the genetic structure of cells. For example, Epstein-Barr virus is involved in the development of Burkitt's lymphoma, Herpes simplex in the development of cervical cancer, and Helicobacter pylori in the development of gastric cancer.

Genetics: About 5% of cancers have a family background.

Age: The older a person is, the more years he or she will be exposed to carcinogens.

Hormonal factors: Hormonal sensitivity increases the risk of neoplasms in tissues such as the breast, endometrium, prostate, ovaries, testes, and thyroid that are sensitive to the hormone. The role of diethylstilbestrol in vaginal carcinoma is well known. Oral contraceptives and long-term estrogen replacement therapy increase the risk of hepatocellular and breast cancer and reduce the risk of ovarian and endometrial cancer.

Nutrition: Foods that increase the risk of cancer include: fat, alcohol, salty meats, foods containing nitrite and nitrate, and high-calorie foods. Foods that reduce the risk of cancer include: High-fiber foods (especially cruciferous vegetables) Such as broccoli, cauliflower, kale), foods containing carotene (carrots, tomatoes, spinach, apricots, peaches, dark green and yellow vegetables) and foods containing vitamins E, C, zinc and selenium. Obesity is also a risk factor. Increases cancers such as postmenopausal breast, colon, kidney and gallbladder cancers.

Immune system: A healthy immune system can detect cancer cells and kill them before they can grow uncontrollably. They increase the risk of cancer.

Prevention

Prevention is done at three levels (the first two levels are very important):

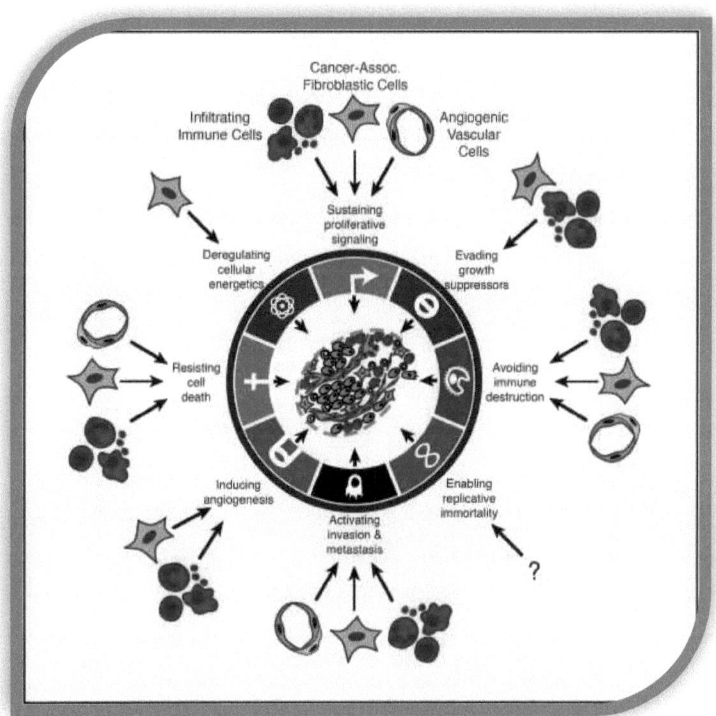

Figure 33. Accessories to the Crime: Functions of Cells Recruited to the Tumor Microenvironment

Primary prevention: Focuses on lifestyle changes to prevent or reduce exposure to carcinogens.

Eating a healthier diet, exercising, reducing exposure to sunlight, and modifying sexual activity are all activities at this level of prevention.

Secondary prevention: Early detection that detects the disease before the manifestations appear. Screening is at this level of prevention. Breast and testicular self-examination, mammography, rectal examination with two fingers (rectal luggage), smear test, blood Stool secretion (OB) and blood test for prostate specific antigen (PSA) help in early detection of cancers. Screening criteria are as follows:

The population should be screened for cancer.

The disease must be detectable in the pre-demonstration stage.

If the disease is diagnosed after the manifestations, it has a bad and unfavorable prognosis

In case of early diagnosis, there is an effective treatment for these diseases.

There is an effective test for screening.

The potential benefits and benefits of screening outweigh the potential risks and costs.

The American Cancer Society has made recommendations for early detection of asymptomatic cancers in high-risk individuals:

In women 29-30 years old, breast self-examination (BSE) and clinical breast examination (CBE) are performed every three years. From the age of 40 onwards, monthly BSE and annual CBE and mammography should also be performed annually.

In women from the age of 21 or 3 years after the start of sexual activity, pelvic exams and Pap smears should be performed annually, and after the age of 30, if Pap smears are normal three times in a row, it may be done every 2-3 years thereafter. And perform an HPV test instead.

Men over the age of 50 (40-45 years for high-risk individuals) should have a PSA test and rectal luggage tested annually.

For men and women over the age of 50, OB (annually) should be performed with flexible sigmoidoscopy (every 5 years) or colonoscopy (every 10 years) or barium enema (every 5 years).

Tertiary prevention: includes care and rehabilitation of patients after cancer diagnosis and treatment.

Grade and stages of cancer

Grading indicates the difference between cancer cells and their progenitor cells. Grades 1 and 2 are well differentiated from normal cells and therefore have a better prognosis. Grades 3 and 4 are less differentiated and much different from normal cells. They look abnormal. These tumors have a worse prognosis.

Grading indicates the extent of primary tumor development (T), tumor involvement to adjacent lymph nodes (N), and metastasis to distant regions (M).

TX: The primary tumor cannot be examined.

T0: There is no evidence of a primary tumor.

TIS: The tumor is in a confined space (Insit).

T1, T2, T3, T4: The size of the tumor increases and the tumor spreads to adjacent areas.

NX: Local lymph nodes cannot be examined.

N0: There is no invasion of the lymph nodes in the area.

N1, N2, N3: Lymph node involvement increases.

MX: Metastasis cannot be detected.

M0: There is no metastasis to distant areas.

M1: There is metastasis.

Cancer diagnosis

The first step in the diagnosis process is to get a complete history and physical examination. The diagnosis of cancer is made by looking at malignant cells in the tumor tissue and under a microscope (a sample obtained from biochemistry or surgery). Various blood tests can be used to help diagnose cancer.

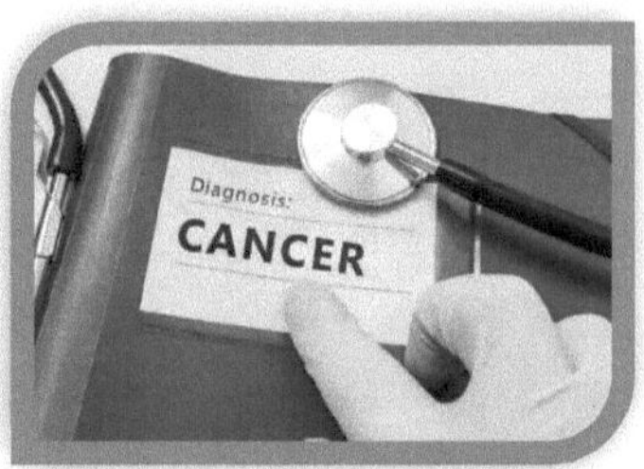

Figure 34. Cancer diagnosis

Some routine tests, such as CBC and its differential count, are not able to detect specific types of cancer, but can show non-specific problems such as anemia and can be used to monitor for cancer side effects. Tumor indicators such as PSA they can also help diagnose cancer and show how effective the treatment.

Cancer treatment methods and their nursing care

Therapies are selected based on the type of tumor, the extent of the disease, the client's underlying diseases, and the client's current condition. Cancer is more effective. For example, they may surgically remove the tumor mass as much as possible and then shrink the residue with chemotherapy.

A) Surgery

Two common approaches to treating primary tumors are: local incision and large incision. Local incision is used when the mass is small and involves removing the mass with a small amount of the marginal edge of the available natural tissue. Large or radical incision. These include the removal of the primary tumor, lymph nodes, adjacent involved structures, and connective tissues that may be at high risk for tumor spread.

Surgery may also have a preventative aspect, that is, tissue with non-vital organs involved in which the possibility of cancerous growth is removed. Presence of family history and genetic predisposition, presence or absence of symptoms, possibility of risk or benefit, ability to detect cancer in early stages and Acceptance of postoperative outcomes by the patient is one of the determining factors for choosing prophylactic surgery. These surgeries include colectomy, mastectomy, and oophorectomy. For example, patients with familial polyposis have a 50% risk of developing colon cancer by age 40, and a 100% risk of developing colon cancer by age 70. There is, therefore, surgery (colectomy) may be necessary for them. Due to the unknown physiological and long-term psychological complications, this type of surgery is used only in special cases.

Relief surgery is another type of surgery that aims to make the patient as comfortable as possible and to improve his satisfaction and make his life more productive. This surgery is used in the following cases:

- ❖ Reduce pain through amputation of nerve endings or implantation of pain control pumps.
- ❖ Removal of obstructions in the respiratory, urinary and gastrointestinal tract.
- ❖ Relieve the pressure on the brain or spinal cord.
- ❖ Prevention of bleeding.
- ❖ Removal of infectious tumors and ulcers.
- ❖ Drain abscesses.

Reconstructive surgery is another form of surgery that is more acceptable for improving function or achieving cosmetic effects. This surgery is used for cancers of the breast, neck and skin.

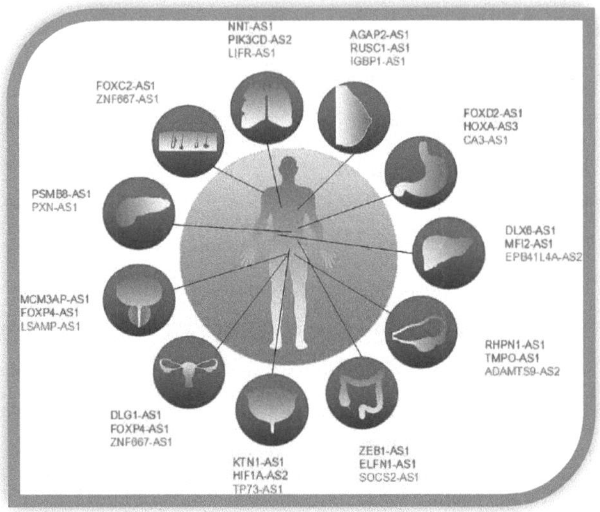

Figure 35. The regulatory role of antisense in cancer

B) Radiotherapy (radiation therapy)

Radiotherapy is the use of high-energy ionizing radiation that destroys the cell's DNA by delaying meiosis and apoptosis, destroying the cell's ability to reproduce. Cells with high dividing power (bone marrow, gastrointestinal tract, lymphatic tissue, Hair cells and sex cells) are more vulnerable to radiation.

In addition to acting on DNA, radiation also causes the formation of free radicals, resulting in a complex chain of chemical reactions in the extracellular fluid. Oxygen radicals formed during the ionization process are easily absorbed by molecules. Adjacent interactions have been shown to kill cells. Tumors with more arteries and higher oxygen delivery are more sensitive to radiation therapy.

Radiation therapy may be used to definitively treat certain cancers, such as Hodgkin's disease, thyroid carcinoma, and cervical cancer, or to control malignancies. It is used to prevent leukemia infiltration into the brain or spinal cord. Palliative radiotherapy is used to alleviate metastatic symptoms, especially when the cancer has spread to the bone marrow and soft tissue, or to treat oncological emergencies such as superior vena cava syndrome. Radiotherapy is used in two ways:

Radiotherapy with external beams (Tele therapy): In this method, the radiation is emitted from a source that is located at a distance from the target area. Radiation is released by high-energy or gamma-ray-producing devices (such as linear accelerators, cobalt, betatron, or radioisotope-containing devices). The most important advantage of high-energy radiation is that the skin is not exposed to radiation.

Therefore, these radiations will have the maximum possible effect when the tumor is deep in the body. Some medical centers treat low-oxygen tumors and radiation-resistant tumors with fine radiation. Like neutrons, it facilitates heavy ions and ions into tissue and destroys target cells along with the cells in its path.

Internal radiotherapy: In this method, radioactive isotopes are implanted directly inside or near the tumor (brachytherapy) or released into the systemic bloodstream.

The two main types of internal radiotherapy are

- ❖ Radiotherapy with coated source 2) Radiotherapy with uncoated source. Radiotherapy with a coated source: It is used as an intermediate or intra-cavity implant. In intracavitary therapy, a radioisotope element (usually cesium-137 or radium-226) is inserted into the applicator and then inserted into the cavity for a specified period of time (24-72 hours). This method is widely used to treat cervical and cervical cancers. In this procedure, the patient must rest (to prevent the instrument from moving into the cavity) and a urinary catheter is inserted to ensure that the bladder is empty. Low residue and an antidiarrheal drug such as diphenoxylate are used. In the interstitial type, selective radioisotopes are implanted inside a needle, bead, bead, tape, or catheter and then implanted directly into the tumor. In this method, the device used is removed less than its place. In coated source radiotherapy, the radioisotope is placed inside a non-radioactive device so that it cannot circulate inside the client's body and contaminate his urine, sweat, blood, and vomit contents, so that the client's secretions and feces are not radioactive. Uncovered source radiotherapy: In this procedure, the radioisotope is circulated throughout the client's body so that the client's urine, sweat, blood, and vomit contents contain the radioactive isotope. In this method, radioisotopes are used intravenously, orally or by direct injection into the body cavities. For example, iodine 131 is used in very low doses and orally to treat Graves' disease and in high doses to treat thyroid cancer.

Safety standards related to radiotherapy

The greater the distance from the radiation source, the lower the contact with the dose of ionizing radiation will be. In other words, the intensity of the radiation is inversely proportional to the square of the distance from the radiation source. For example, if you are standing 4 feet away from the radiation source, you will be contacted with the amount of radiation received at a distance of 2 feet.

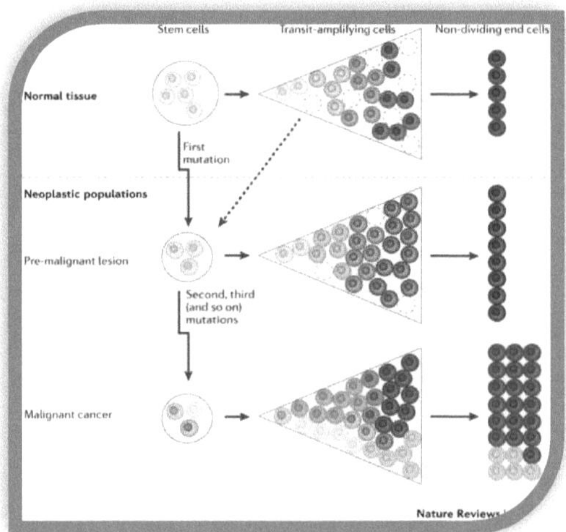

Figure 36. Cancer stem cell definitions and terminology

98

When caring for a client who has implants inside the uterus, to be less exposed to radiation, you should stand on the client's bed instead of next to him. The minimum distance from the radiation source should be 6 feet (180 cm). The duration of exposure to the radiation source during an 8-hour shift should be limited to 30 minutes of direct care of the client.

Client care among nursing staff Each shift should be done in rotation to limit the proximity of each staff to the radiation source. Pregnant nurses should not care for clients receiving radiotherapy. The use of lead protective coatings reduces radiation exposure, although its use is cumbersome for nurses. Clients who have an indoor radioactive implant with a covered source should use a private room, bathroom and toilet. Or is considered a staircase. In their room, there should always be a pair of long-hand forceps and a serum chamber called a pig, so that if a radiation source leaves the body, it can be removed using forceps and placed inside the pig. Clients receiving radiotherapy with an uncovered source also need a private room, bathroom and toilet. They should be taught to pull the siphon several times after each use of the toilet. Their food is served on disposable plates and dishes.

Bed linen and rubbish are stored in the room until discharge from the room. Caregivers must put on a new pair of shoes each time they enter the room so that the radioactive isotope does not get out of the room. Gloves should be used to move or move body fluids. In prostate brachytherapy, there is a possibility of others coming into contact with a small number of radiation beams. These beams of radiation have little penetration, but the client must use a condom during intercourse in the first few weeks after brachytherapy. Also, within two months. First, avoid close contact (less than 6 feet) with pregnant women and young children for more than 5 minutes a day.

Some notes

The dose of radiation is determined in terms of unitity (Gray). Each dose is equal to 100 Rad (Rad). Increasing the dose increases the side effects. In addition, the received dose of radiation in therapeutic use is more than soothing cases. Only the area that is being treated in the area is affected by radiation, so complications such as hair loss occur only in that area. Radiotherapy with direct doses is better than single doses because it gives less side effects due to giving the opportunity to repair normal cells and on the other hand it is more effective because it is possible that tumor cells are in one of the vulnerable phases of the cell cycle during treatment.

Side effects of radiotherapy

Skin reactions and fatigue are among the common complications of radiotherapy that are not related to the body area being treated with radiotherapy. The patient should be educated about skin care in the treated area:

- ❖ Keep your skin dry.
- ❖ Refrain from washing the area until it is not allowed, and when it is allowed to be washed, gently rinse the skin with a mild soap and put a towel on the area to dry the skin. Remove from cold or lukewarm water to wash.
- ❖ Clear lines or marks that have been inked on the skin.
- ❖ Do not use powder, lotion, cream and deodorant in the area.
- ❖ Use loose clothing in that area to prevent friction and wear of clothing with the skin in that area. To shave the hair in the area, use electric razors. Do not use special lotions before and after shaving.
- ❖ Avoid contact of the skin of the area with direct sunlight, swimming pools containing chlorine, hot water or ice.

Specific manifestations related to different areas of the body in addition to skin manifestations include: mucocytes, zerostomia (dry mouth), tooth decay, esophagitis, dysphagia, nausea and vomiting, diarrhea, tenesmus (painful and fruitless pressure to pass stool or urine) Inflammation of the bladder and urethra, alopecia and bone marrow suppression. All of these complications are either due to acute changes caused by inflammation or are caused by chronic changes associated with fibrosis. Women of childbearing age may experience permanent or temporary infertility.

During radiotherapy, CBC is usually done once a week to check the degree of bone marrow suppression.

Strategies for controlling side effects are similar to those for controlling the side effects of chemotherapy, which will be described below.

Chemotherapy: Chemotherapy drugs kill cancer cells by affecting the cell cycle.

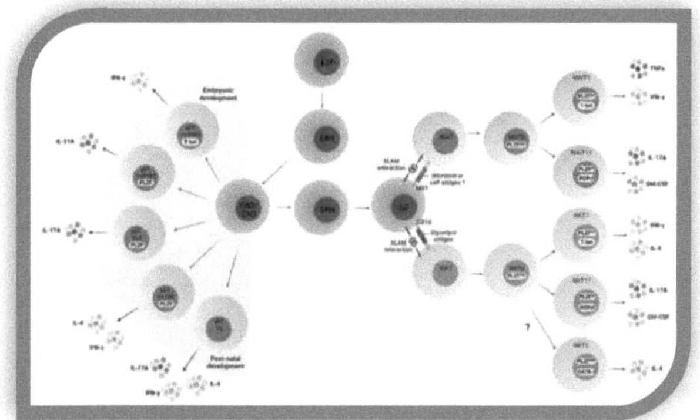

Figure 37. Regulation and Functions of Protumoral Unconventional T Cells

Cell cycle stages

Phase G_0: This phase is a period of time in which the cell is at rest and cell division does not occur. This phase continues until a trigger message activates phase G_1.

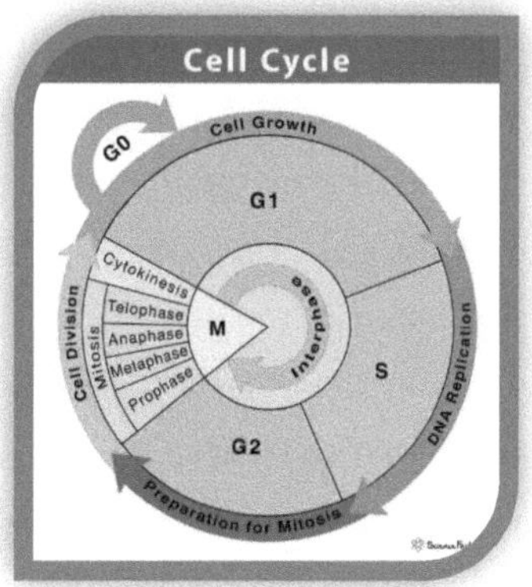

Figure 38. Cell cycle

Phase G₂: In this phase, which lasts 8 hours or more, protein and ribonucleic acid are synthesized. In phase G₁, there is a stage called the inhibitory point, and the cell progresses to phase S after reaching this stage. The cell begins DNA synthesis 1-3 hours after passing the inhibitory point. Acquiring the ability to begin the process of DNA synthesis marks the end of the G₁ phase.

Phase S: The synthesis of proteins and DNA belonging to new chromosomes takes place in this phase, which takes about 6-8 hours.

Phase G: In this phase, a series of biochemical processes, including RNA synthesis, take place to prepare the cell for mitosis. This goose lasts between 2-5 hours.

Phase M1: which is the stage of mitosis and two sister cells are formed.

Types of chemotherapy drugs

The most important classes of chemotherapy drugs are:

- ❖ *Alkylating agents:* such as cisplatin, cyclophosphamide, mustard nitrogen, and melphalans. These drugs change the structure of DNA and overlap DNA strands. Inflammation of the tongue, alopecia, genital suppression, and renal toxicity (especially cisplatin) were noted.

- ❖ *Anti-metabolites:* such as cytarabine, 5-fluorouracil, methotrexate, mercaptopurine, etc. These drugs are specific to the cell cycle in stage S, ie they interfere with protein and DNA synthesis. Nausea and vomiting, diarrhea, bone marrow suppression, inflammation of the anus and tongue, kidney poisoning (especially in methotrexate) and liver poisoning are the most important side effects of these drugs.

- ❖ *Antitumor antibiotics:* such as bleomycin, danurobicin, doxorubicin (adriamycin). These drugs that interfere with RNA and DNA synthesis have side effects such as bone marrow depression, nausea and vomiting, severe alopecia, anorexia and intoxication. Danurobicin and doxorubicin).

* ***Vinca (herbal) alkaloids:*** such as vincristine and vinblastine, which are specific for cell cycle in stage M. Bone marrow depression, neuropathy and inflammation of the tongue (especially the use of vincristine) are side effects of these drugs.

* ***Hormonal factors:*** such as androgens and anti-androgens, estrogens and antiestrogens, steroids, etc. Depending on the type of drug, the side effects are different.

Note: Salvage therapy is a form of treatment used for cases of cancer recurrence and when the disease has not responded to standard treatment. This method uses a combination of cisplatin and cytarabine in high doses as well as dexamethasone. Feverish neutropenia and hemorrhage are the most important complications of this treatment. In general, the goal of this treatment is mainly greater comfort and increase life expectancy.

Ways of prescribing chemotherapy drugs: The amount of chemotherapy drug depends on the patient's entire body surface, the patient's previous response to radiation and chemotherapy, and the function of vital organs.

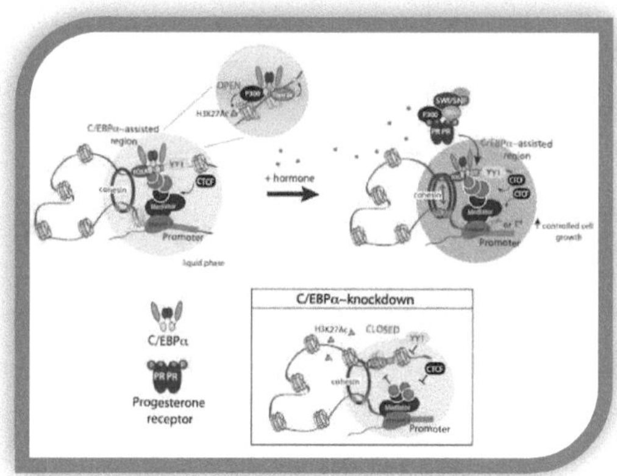

Figure 39. Growth inhibitory effect of progestins on breast cancer cells

The prescribed dose enters the body through various routes such as intravenous, oral, subcutaneous and intramuscular. Chemotherapy involves regional, intra-arterial, intra-cavity, intraperitoneal and intrathecal.

Intravenous chemotherapy: Care should be taken in the selection of the vessel and the technique of inserting the needle into the vessel. Among the peripheral arteries, the large vessels of the fleshy and soft forearms take precedence over the other vessels. Should not be used for injection.

The lower extremities and distal areas of the area that were last used for injection, as well as the vessels in the back of the hand and the vessels in the flexed area (such as the wrist or elbow) are not suitable for injection. Intravenous chemotherapy is the most common type Chemotherapy is given to the patient's body and it is better to use scalp vein for injection.

Before and after chemotherapy and at intervals, the vessel should be flushed with normal saline solution. When prescribing intravenous chemotherapy drugs, the nurse should be careful of leakage of the drug from the vessel, especially in the form of vesicants. Nitrogen mustard, vin blastin, vincristine, vindsin and mitomycin are blistering drugs. If these drugs enter the subcutaneous tissue, they cause tissue necrosis and damage to ligaments, nerves and adjacent blood vessels. The vessels include: no return of blood from the intravenous catheter, resistance to fluid flow into the vein and swelling, pain or redness of the site.

In case of drug leakage, do the following
- ❖ Stop injecting the medicine immediately.
- ❖ Apply a cold compress on the area. The use of ice and cold compresses on the area of Vinca alkaloids is prohibited.
- ❖ Tell your doctor. Your doctor may aspiration the remaining medicine through a tube, needle, and injection site. He or she may also inject antibodies (sodium thiosulfate, hyaluronidase, and sodium bicarbonate).
- ❖ Never apply pressure directly to the position by hand.

❖ Examine the area regularly for pain, redness, swelling, bulging, and necrosis.

❖ Record the appearance of the area before and after chemotherapy.

An allergic reaction is another complication that is more likely with drugs such as cisplatin, carboplatin, and L-aspartase. If an allergic reaction occurs, do the following:

❖ Stop injecting medicine immediately.

❖ Keep the airway open.

❖ Inform the doctor.

❖ Keep the intravenous route open by injecting normal saline.

❖ Place the client in an open arch position and raise the legs.

❖ Check vital signs every two minutes until the client's condition stabilizes.

❖ Use epinephrine, aminophylline, diphenhydramine and corticosteroids as directed by your doctor.

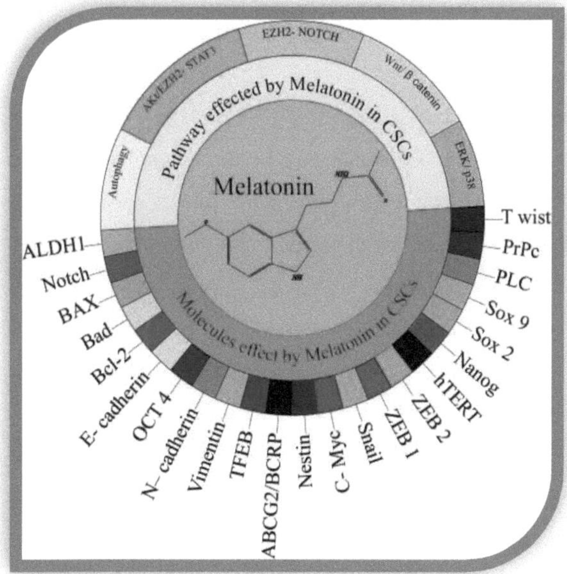

Figure 40. Targeting cancer stem cells by melatonin: Effective therapy for cancer treatment

Regional chemotherapy: To treat radiation keratosis, fluorescein creams are used topically. The intraperitoneal method is used especially for cancers of the abdomen, such as ovarian cancer. The intracavitary method is suitable for areas such as the abdomen, bladder and side. And the intrathecal method is suitable for CNS tumors because most drugs that are used systemically cannot cross the blood-brain barrier.

The concept of cancer

Cancer is probably the disease that most people are most afraid of, the word cancer itself scares people a lot, and most people think the death toll is much higher (Boris, Mirowitz, Kerry, and Murrow), 1987; quoted by Sarafino, 2008). Cancer is a deadly disease because no effective cure has been found for it. Every year in the world, thousands of people die from this disease (Asimov, 2003). Cancer is a dangerous disease that produces sores and swellings inside or outside the body, similar to crab legs, and for this reason it is called cancer in Persian, but in medicine it is called "cancer". This name is used in pathology for any disorder and also refers to cellular and tissue chaos.

Cancer is generally called the abnormal growth of cells in the body. In other words, any internal and external factor that disrupts the natural mechanism of the body organs and causes that organ to grow irregularly, causes cancer (Pourkazemi, 2003). We know that our bodies are made of cells, and during each person's life, physical growth is caused by cell division in most tissues, and it is only through this mechanism that every living thing constantly wears out its damaged cells with new cells. It replaces and keeps its texture working, and this is a systematic process. But when the phenomenon of cell division goes out of its normal course, it causes a large mass of tissue called a tumor. Tumors are of two types, benign and malignant, a malignant tumor attacks healthy tissues, while benign tumors do not develop and hence malignant tumors are cancerous.

Cancer cells can come out of the tumor and spread through the bloodstream; these cells settle in other parts of the body and begin to grow and multiply, producing other tumors. The movement of cancer cells and their transfer to other parts of the body is called metastasis. Tumors eventually destroy vital organs and cause death (Asimov, 2003). But despite the deadly and incurable disease, if every human being uses a proper and healthy diet and avoids environmental risk factors, which are very important, it is very easy to observe these two very important parameters, the risk of a deadly disease is very high. Decreases (Pourkazemi, 2003).

One of the basic characteristics of life and growth is that cells proliferate under controlled and specific conditions. Scientists know what the natural pattern of tissue growth is (Gaiton, 1985; quoted in Sarafino, 2008). Irregularities in this process cause the cells to grow indefinitely, which usually leads to the formation of a gland called a neoplasm (tumor) (AMA, 1989; Tortora and Grabowski, 1993; quoted in Sarafino, 2008). Although we know little about the process that keeps the number of different cells in the body at a certain level, researchers have discovered an enzyme that is abundant in glandular cells and is likely to cause these cells to proliferate. Kanter, Hirt, Bachetti, and Harley, 1994; quoted in Sarafino, 2008). Some neoplasms are harmless or benign, but some are malignant (Sarafino, 2008).

Cancer is a disease of cells characterized by the indefinite proliferation of cells that make up malignant neoplasms. Although there are more than 200 types of cancer, major cancers are divided into four types (Nelson, 1989; Tortora and Grabowski, 1993; Williams, 1990; quoted in Sarafino, 2008). These four types are:

Carcinoma: A malignant neoplasm of skin cells and cells that cover many organs in the body, such as the gastrointestinal tract, genitals, and respiratory tract. About 85% of human cancers are carcinomas.

Lymphoma: or cancers of the lymphatic system.

Sarcoma: A malignant neoplasm of connective tissue such as bone, muscle, or connective tissue.

Leukemia: or cancer of the blood components, such as bone marrow, which leads to overproduction of white blood cells (Sarafino, 2008; Curtis, 2003).

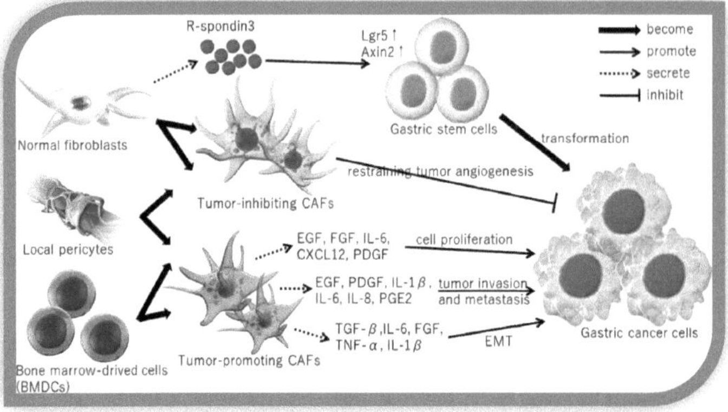

Figure 41. Tumor microenvironment in gastric cancers - Oya - 2020 - Cancer Science

The prevalence of cancer

In 1991, it was reported that there are 6 million new cancer patients worldwide each year, and that one-tenth of all deaths are from cancer (Agden, 1996; cited by Curtis, 2003). In the United Kingdom, cancers and coronary heart disease are the leading cause of death, and these chronic diseases account for half of all deaths (Curtis, 2003).

Mortality rates of cancer disability are alarming. Cancer kills more than 520,000 Americans each year, and 1.3 million new cases are diagnosed. About half of people who get Mitella cancer can expect to live more than 5 years. Although cancer may spread throughout the body, since 1950, almost all increases in cancer mortality have been due to neoplasms (tumors) of one part of the body, the lungs (Sarafino, 2008).

Cancer Effects

What are the physical effects of cancer and how does it cause death? Cancer spreads to different parts of the body, and its growth in each part interferes with normal growth and function there. As the disease progresses, it causes pain, mostly due to pressure on normal tissues and nerves or obstruction of body fluid flow (Malzak and Wall, 1982; quoted in Sarafino, 2008). Severe pain affects 40% of people with moderate to severe cancer and 70% to 90% of those with advanced cancer (Foley, 1985; Greenwald, Bonica, & Berger, 1987; Ward et al., 1993; Sarafino, 2008). This disease directly and indirectly leads to death. In its direct form, the cancer spreads over time to sensitive organs such as the brain, liver or lungs. And it competes with those organs to get the nutrients it needs, causing tissue death. Cancer kills in two indirect ways; Either self-illness weakens the sufferer, or both illness and treatment reduce the appetite and the body's ability to fight infection (Laszlo, 1987; quoted in Sarafino, 2008).

Prognosis and causes of cancer

The prognosis of cancer depends on how early the cancer and its location are diagnosed (ACS, 1966; Batista and Graver, 1988; Laszlo, 1987; Williams, 1990; quoted in Sarafino, 2008). Cancer is as likely to be a specific disease with a single, unknown cause as bleeding or heart failure. Cancer is a type of change in cell behavior in response to several harmful factors, some of which are known and some are not (Wingit, 1994).

Cancer is caused by the interaction of genetic and environmental factors, and stress can play a stimulating role in the development and spread of this disease. Environmental factors include smoking, diet type, UV rays, and the presence of hazardous substances at work and at home. Some researchers have found a link between viral and the development of some cancers, such as liver and cervix (Laszlo, 1987; Williams, 1990; quoted by Sarafino, 2008). In cervical cancer, the transmission of the virus is likely to occur during sexual intercourse. Because not all women who come in contact with viruses get this cancer, it seems that the effect of the infection depends on environmental and genetic factors or is associated with them to lead to the disease (Sarafino, 2008).

Age, gender and socio-cultural factors in cancer

The risk of cancer usually increases with age, especially after middle age. In all types of cancer, the incidence of the disease quadruples from the age of 40 to 80 (Moore et al., 1985; quoted by Sarfino, 2008).

The risk of developing cancer among Americans is related to gender. Apart from skin cancer, the most common cancers recently diagnosed are prostate cancer in men, and breast cancer in women, and for both sexes, lung and colorectal cancer (ACS, 1996; quoted in Sarfino, 2008). In the UK, too, there appear to be gender differences in cancer mortality: women are more vulnerable to breast cancer (20% mortality rate), and men are more susceptible to lung cancer (36% mortality rate). While the incidence of cancer-related deaths does not appear to be increasing, the incidence of lung cancer in women has steadily increased over the past few years, in part due to declining smoking in It is among men (Curtis, 2003).

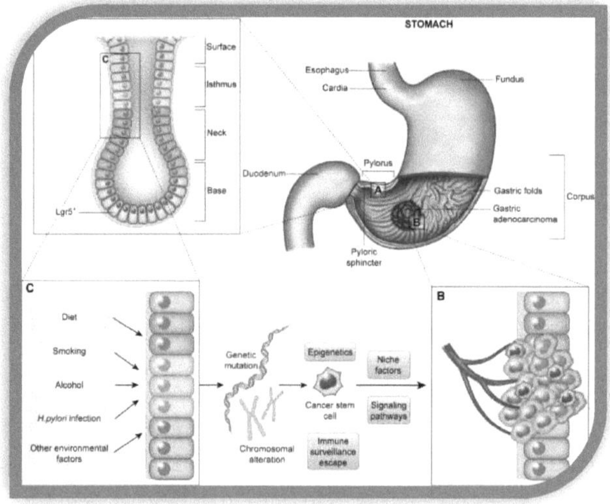

Figure 42. Helicobacter pylori infection and gastric cancer biology: tempering a double-edged sword

The link between cancer and socio-cultural factors is evident in mortality data from different ethnic groups in the United States. Among men and women, the rate of cancer deaths for blacks is twice that of Asian Americans, Native Americans, and Hispanics, and the rate of white deaths is intermediate (USDHHS, 1995; quoted by Sarfino, 2008). Although the incidence of cancer is not so different between blacks and whites, black cancer is usually diagnosed later (ACS, 1996; Eli et al., 1994; quoted by Sarfino, 2008). There are also national differences in cancer prevalence. Lung cancer, for example, is more common in the United Kingdom than in Nigeria, and gastric cancer is more common in Japan than in Uganda (AMA, 1989; quoted in Sarfino, 2008).

Diagnosis and treatment of cancer

By recognizing the signs of cancer risk and having regular tests, you can increase the chance of early detection of cancer. The process of diagnosing cancer consists of three stages (AMA, 1989; Laszlo, 1987; Nguyen et al., 1994; cited in Sarafino, 2008): First, performing a blood or urine test to detect the presence of cancer, or detecting early signs of Such as abnormal amounts of hormones or enzymes. Second: X-ray images or other methods that help the doctor see the structure of the internal organs and examine the mass. Third, the doctor removes a small piece of suspicious tissue, performs a biopsy or biopsy. Even when the tissue is deep in the abdomen, it can usually be sampled with minor surgery and local anesthesia. The ideal goal in cancer treatment is to cure the patient, that is, to completely get rid of the cancer.

Achieving this desirable goal is possible when all parts of the cancer are found and eliminated (Gaiton, 1985; Laszlo, 1987; quoted in Sarafino, 2008). If all the cancerous tissue is not destroyed, the symptoms may disappear for a while and come back after a while. Sometimes, doctors make evidence that all cancerous tissue is gone, but often this is not certain. This is why they use the 5-year survival rate as an indicator of treatment success. There are generally three types of cancer treatments: surgery, radiation therapy, and chemotherapy that are used alone or together. In choosing the type of treatment, the patient and the physician consider several factors, such as the size and location of the tumor, whether or not it has metastasized, and the effect of treatment on the patient's quality of life. The factor that sometimes inappropriately affects the choice of treatment is the patient's age (Sarafino, 2008).

Surgery: From a medical point of view, surgery is usually the preferred treatment for eliminating malignancies such as breast or colorectal cancer (Laszlo, 1987; Williams, 990; quoted in Sarafino, 2008). If the cancerous tissue is in one place, surgery alone is often quite effective, and if the tissue has spread, surgery may be effective in removing the large cancerous mass and the rest of the cells must be removed with radiation and chemotherapy. Sometimes, the surgeon removes a large portion of the tissue near the cancerous mass because of the possibility that the cancer may have spread to that area.

Radiation therapy: Radiation therapy in high doses changes the cells of the body in a way that they either die or lose their ability to reproduce (Holam, 1994; quoted by Sarafino, 2008). In the treatment of cancer, radiation therapy is used in two ways (Purish and Liles, 1983; McNaul, 1984; quoted by Sarafino, 2008). External beam therapy involves irradiating strong radiation to malignant tissue for a few seconds or minutes. This method is more common than others and people consider this method when they hear the term "radiation therapy". External beam therapy is usually given several times a week and may last for weeks. The second method of treatment with internal radiation is to place a radioactive substance surgically or by injection, in the body, near or inside the mass. Although radiation therapy is painless, it can have unpleasant and problematic side effects. These complications depend on the location of the cancer and the amount of radiation. Because radiation therapy affects both malignant and healthy cells, the site of radiation exposure may cause sores, burns, and hair loss. Also, especially if the area undergoing radiation therapy is large or in the abdomen, the person may experience nausea, vomiting, loss of appetite, infertility, and decreased bone marrow activity (Sarafino, 2008).

Chemotherapy: In chemotherapy, patients take strong oral or injectable drugs that circulate throughout the body and kill rapidly proliferating cells (Boris and Lyles, 1983; Laszlo, 1987; Williams, 1990; quoted in Sarafino, 2008). Of course, the target is cancer cells, most of which multiply rapidly. Some types of cancer respond better to current drugs than others. Testicular cancers and types of leukemia respond very well, but not cancers of the brain and pancreas. One of the problems with chemotherapy is that the drugs available also kill certain types of natural cells that divide rapidly; Such as bone marrow cells, covering the mouth and gastrointestinal tract, and hair follicles, especially on the head. Some chemotherapy regimens last a long time and cause many side effects, including decreased immunity to infection, mouth ulcers, hair loss, nausea and vomiting, and damage to internal organs. AMA, 1989; USDHHS, 1983; Williams, 1990; quoted by Sarafino, 2008).

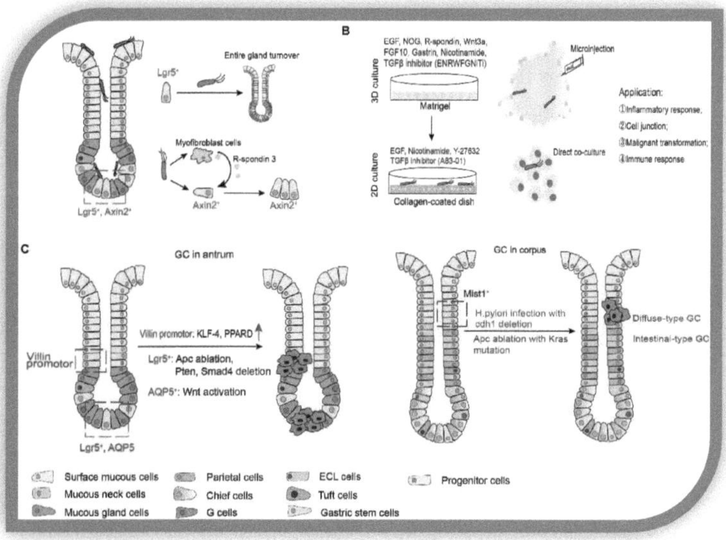

Figure 43. Frontiers, Gastric Stem Cells: Physiological and Pathological Perspectives

For many patients, the most excruciating side effects of chemotherapy are nausea and vomiting, which patients experience during and immediately after treatment. (Sarafino, 2008). Cancer treatment is not only unpleasant but can also be complex and tedious. Most cancer patients have to take medication at home, and many have to go to the hospital regularly for tests, eat certain foods, or change their diet and other daily habits. Due to these conditions, it is likely that cancer patients will be very incomplete in their treatment regimen (Sarafino, 2008). Although most adults seem to follow the treatment regimen well, adolescents and minority groups and the lower classes do not. Acceptance of treatment regimens depends on a range of psychosocial factors in an individual's life and is influenced by them (Sarafino, 2008).

The role of psychology in cancer

Although the calming (temporal rather than therapeutic) effect of psychology on cancer was first suggested by Galen in 300-200 AD, it was not until recent that the relationship was systematically studied. It is believed that 85% of potential cancers are preventable. Therefore, the field of psychology has a great share in all stages of the disease. In fact, psychology can be helpful in the first place as a pain reliever in the development of cancer. Cancer cells are present in most people, although not all people get cancer. This suggests that there are individual differences in cancer vulnerability. Lifestyle and other factors may trigger cancer. For example, evidence suggests that there is a strong association between smoking and lung cancer, although not all smokers develop lung cancer. This is in fact a relationship of probability and not cause and effect (Curtis, 2003).

In addition to the above, not all people with cancer show the same progression to death. It can be said that psychology plays an important role in limiting the spread of cancer. Likewise, not all people who suffer from cancer die from cancer. Psychology may even play a role in increasing life expectancy after cancer (Curtis, 2003). Behavior may affect the onset and progression of cancer. For example, Smith and Jacobsen (1989; cited in Curtis, 2003). Report that 30% of cancers are related to tobacco use, 35% to diet, 7% to sexual and reproductive behavior, and 3% to alcohol.

Stress may also play a role in the onset and progression of cancer (Curtis, 2003). Various studies have suggested that cancer may be related to stress. Various studies have shown that infectious diseases increase during stress. Some researchers have even claimed to have identified a "cancer-prone personality" (Carlson, 2007). The effect of stress on cancer depends on several factors such as the type or source of stress, its duration, the person's response to stress and its timing (before or after the onset of cancer). If stress has a causal role in causing cancer, this event has been achieved by disrupting the immune system in the fight against disease and increasing risk behavioral factors such as smoking (Sarafino, 2008).

Other psychological factors that may play a role in cancer include: perceived level of stress on the stressors, coping styles, mild chronic stress (not clinical depression), personality C and low stubbornness profile (Curtis, 2003). Overall, most researchers believe that stress (and personality variables related to stress tolerance) play a greater role in the growth of cancerous glands than their formation (Carlson, 2007).

Psychological responses to cancer

Cancer, like all chronic diseases, involves a series of constantly changing risks and problems that often intensify over time (Sarafino, 2008). Emotional responses to cancer include severe depression, sadness, lack of control, personality change, anger, and anxiety. These conditions occur in more than 20% of patients (Curtis, 2003).

Cancer causes unique stress to the patient and his family. These patients consider cancer their "real killer" and a disease that leads to pain, disability, and deformity. Even among patients who recover and adapt well in the first months or years, there is a fear of recurrence. And if the disease returns, some people become psychologically paralyzed due to fear (Miges, Mendelssohn, 1979; quoted by Sarafino, 2008). In addition, some patients find the treatment more hateful than the disease itself. The rate of cancer acceptance by the individual affects the outcome of treatment and the course of the disease. In people with severe stress and maladaptation, the activity of the immune system is low, and some evidence suggests that if the immune system is impaired, the disease progresses faster (Kikalt-Glasser and Glasser, 1986; Levy et al.,

1985; Red et al., 1991; quoted by Sarafino, 2008). Obvious predictors of emotional responses to cancer include a history of psychiatry, lack of social support, age, and lack of intimacy. In the case of advanced cancer, the patient's psychological health is closely related to their physical health (Pinder et al., 1993; cited by Curtis, 2003). Although it may be very difficult for patients to adjust to cancer in the first months and as the disease progresses, their ability to adapt to the disease increases over time, during the recovery period or after recovery. Borisch, Mirowitz, Kerry and Murrow, 1987; Glans and Lerman, 1992; quoted in Sarafino, 2008). Up to about 2 years after diagnosis, patients' psychosocial function reaches the same level as before diagnosis. Adaptation in cancer patients depends on many aspects of the disease and their psychosocial conditions. For example, patients' attainment of emotional adjustment depends on their age and physical condition middle-aged or older people with more physical disabilities appear to feel much more distressed than older people or those with less disabilities (Wincore, Trit, Winocor-Kaplan and Satariano, 1990; quoted by Sarafino, 2008). Most patients with major depression are those who are completely physically disabled due to illness or pain (Borisch, Mirowitz, Kerry, & Murrow, 1987; Spiegel, Sands, & Kopman, 1994; quoted in Sarafino, 2008). Many cancer patients develop psychological problems that result from changes in their relationships with family and friends. In some cases, the patient may avoid social relationships because he or she feels ugly or embarrassed because of illness, especially if his or her body shape has changed markedly (Megs and Mendelssohn, 1979; quoted in Sarafino, 2008). But the other two causes are probably more common (Bloom, Kang, & Romano, 1991; quoted in Sarafino, 2008).

First, his physical condition and treatment of the disease may prevent him from meeting others. Second, people may distance themselves from the individual. Although this problem sometimes occurs due to fear and ignorance, for example, when people think that cancer is contagious, but sometimes there are other causes (Sarafino, 2008). In addition to emotional responses to cancer, cognitive responses suggest that having a "fighting spirit" is negatively related to anxiety and depression (i.e., a strong "fighting spirit" eliminates anxiety and depression). The reason why this happens is not known, although the biological psychological-social model of health discussed earlier may provide answers in this regard (Curtis, 2003).

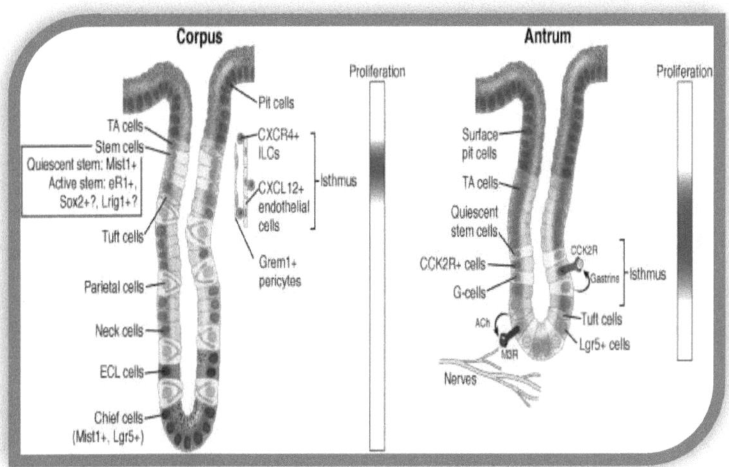

Figure 44. The Origins of Gastric Cancer From Gastric Stem Cells: Lessons From Mouse Models

Psychosocial interventions for cancer

Efforts to help the individual cope with the disease begin at the time of the diagnostic interview (Roberts et al., 1994; quoted in Sarafino, 2008). Positive adaptation to the disease increases when he or she is conscious, his or her spouse, or another influential person is present, allows the person to express their feelings, and then expresses information about the prognosis and types of treatment (Sarafino, 2008). To increase the individual's adaptation to the disease and improve the quality of life, several types of psychosocial interventions have been used successfully (Mir and Mark, 1995; quoted in Sarafino, 2008). The focus of these methods has been to help reduce nausea from chemotherapy (Kerry and Borisch, 1988; quoted in Sarafino, 2008). The two methods that help the patient the most are: relaxation training and regular desensitization.

Other therapeutic interventions have focused on a wider range of issues and have shown that psychosocial methods not only increase the adjustment of individuals, but also increase their chances of survival (Sarafino, 2008).

Because of the social problems that cancer patients face, they and their families benefit from family therapy and participation in support groups that include group education and discussion (Helgson and Cohen, 1996; Tavian, 1991; Quoted from Sarafino, 2008). The American Cancer Society runs about 3,000 local centers that offer a variety of services, including rehabilitation programs and support groups for patients, some of which focus on a specific type of cancer or help families whose children have cancer. Laszlo, 1987; quoted by Sarafino, 2008).

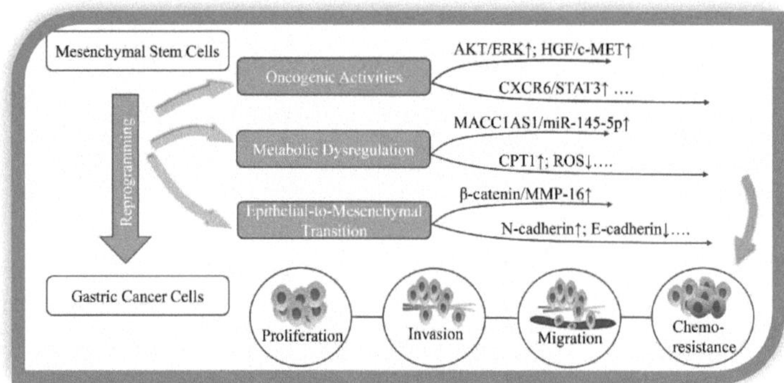

Figure 45. Frontiers, Mesenchymal Stem Cells in Gastric Cancer: Vicious but Hopeful

References

[1]. Siegel R, Nailshadham D, Ahmedin, J. Cancer statistics, 2012. CA Cancer J Clin; 2012. 62(1): 10- 29.

[2]. oore MA, Eser S, Igisinov N, Igisinov S, Mohagheghi M, Jarrahi AM, et al. Cancer Epidemiology and Control in North-Western and Central Asia - Past, Present and Future. Asian Pac J Cancer Prev; 2010. 11(Suppl 2): 17-32.

[3]. Zendehdel K, Sedighi Z, Hassanloo J, Nahvijou A. Improving Quality of Cancer Registration in Iran. Part1: Evaluation and Comparison of Cancer Registration Results in the Country. Hakim Res J; 2010. 12: 42-48. (Persian)

[4]. Berek JS. Berek and Novak's gynecology. 14th ed. Philadelphia: Lippincott Williams & Wilkins, 2007.

[5]. Stewart SL, King JB, Thompson TD, Friedman C, Wingo PA. Cancer mortality surveillance-united states, 1990-2000. MMWR Surveill Summ; 2004. 53(3): 1-108.

[6]. Baig S, Ali TS. Evaluation of efficacy of self-breast examination for breast cancer prevention: a cost effective screening tool. Asian Pac J Cancer Prev; 2006. 7(1):154 -6.

[7]. Jalalvandi M, Khodadoostan M. Married womwn and PAP SMEAR, what they know? How they do? Iran J Nurs; 2005. 18 (41&42): 139-144

[8]. Van Laarhoven HW, Schilderman J, Verhagen CA, Vissers KC, Prins J. Perspectives on death and afterlife in relation to quality of life, depression, and hopelessness in cancer patients without evidence of disease and advanced cancer patients. J Pain Symptom Manage; 2011. 41(6): 1048-59.

[9]. Carter J, Huang H, Chase DM, Walker JL, Cella D, Wenzel L. Sexual function of patients with endometrial cancer enrolled in the Gynecologic Oncology Group LAP2 Study. Int J Gynecol Cancer; 2012. 22(9): 1624-33.

[10]. Akkuzu G, Ayhan A. Sexual Functions of Turkish Women with Gynecologic Cancer during the Chemotherapy Process. Asian Pac J Cancer Prev; 2013. 14(6): 3561-64.

[11]. Aarstad HJ, Heimdal JH, Aarsta AK, Olofsson J. Personality traits in head and neck squamous cell carcinoma patients in relation to the disease state, disease extent and prognosis. Acta Otolaryngal; 2002. 122(8): 892-99.

[12]. Ogden J. Health Psychology. Translated by Kachuie M. Tehran: Arjmand. 2016. (Persian)

[13]. Nakaya N, Hansen PE, Schapiro IR, Eplov LF, Saito-Nakaya K, Uchitomi Y. Et al. Personality traits and cancer survival: A Danish cohort study. Br J Cancer; 2006. 95(11): 146-152.

[14]. McKenna MC, Zevon MA, Corn B, Rounds J. Psychosocial factors and the development of breast cancer: A meta-analysis. Health Psychol; 1999. 18(5): 520-31.

[15]. Persky VW, Kempthorne-Rawson J, Shekelle RB. Personality and risk of cancer: 20 year follow up of the Western Electric Study. Psychosom Med; 1987. 49(5): 435-449.

[16]. Nakaya N, Tsubono Y, Hosokawa T, Nishino Y, Ohkubo T, Hozawa A. et al. Personality and the risk of cancer. J Natl Cancer Inst; 2003. 95(11): 799-805.

[17]. Whiteside TJ, Hererman RB. The role of natural killer cells in immune surveillance of cancer. Curr Opin Immunol; 1995. 7(5): 704-710

[18]. Garssen B, Goodkin k. On the role of immunological factors as mediators between psychological factors and cancer progression. Psychiatry Res; 1999. 85(1): 51-61.

[19]. Spiegal D, Moore R. Imagery and hypnosis in the treatment of cancer patients. Oncology (Williston Park); 1997. 11(8): 1179-89.

[20]. A Molaei, H Alizadeh Otaghvar, M Tarahomi, D Shojaei, L Mohajerzadeh, M Baghoori, F Niazi, A bizarre presentation of Peutz–jegher's syndrome in a 2 year old, Iranian Journal of Pediatric Surgery, 2017, 3 (2), 104-106

[21]. A Nurmeksela, et al., Relationships between nursing management, nurses' job satisfaction, patient satisfaction, and medication errors at the unit Level: A correlational study. Research Square 2020; 1 (1): 1-22.

[22]. A Rezapour, N Qaderi, S Golalipour, et al., Comparison of the Adhesion Rate of Implant Cemented Coatings with 3 Types of Glass Ionomer Cement, Zinc Phosphate and Resin on Blinds Made of Adhesive Composite after Thermal Stress, Journal of Pharmaceutical Negative Results, 2022, 3304-3316

[23]. A Zeidani, N Qaderi, S Akbari Zavieh, S Golalipour, M Golmohammadi, Cardiovascular outcomes and Dental careof COVID-19: a systematic review and met analysis, Neuro Quantology, 2022, 20(8), 3060-3066

[24]. AAR Ghahroudi, AR Rokn, AR Shamshiri, N Samiei, Does timing of implant placement affect esthetic results in single-tooth implants? A cohort evaluation based on Mpes, Journal of Esthetic and Restorative Dentistry, 32(7), 2020, 715-725

[25]. AR Hosseini Khalili, et al. Angiotensin-converting enzyme genotype and late respiratory complications of mustard gas exposure. BMC Pulm Med. 2008;8(1):15.

[26]. B Mahmoodiyeh, S Etemadi, A Kamali, S Rajabi, M Milanifard, Evaluating the Effect of Different Types of Anesthesia on Intraoperative Blood Glucose Levels in Diabetics and Non-Diabetics Patients: A Systematic Review and Meta-Analysis, Annals of the Romanian Society for Cell Biology, 2021, 2559–2572

[27]. B Shakiba, et al., Medical Workplace Civility Watch: An Attempt to Improve the Medical Training Culture, Journal of Iranian Medical Council, 2022, 5 (1), 227-228

[28]. DH Birman, Investigation of the Effects of Covid-19 on Different Organs of the Body, Eurasian Journal of Chemical, Medicinal and Petroleum Research, 2023, 2 (1), 24-36

[29]. E Ghaibi, et al., Comparison of Marital Satisfaction, Emotional Divorce and Religious Commitment among Nurses and Staff of Ahvaz Government Hospitals, Eurasian Journal of Chemical, Medicinal and Petroleum Research, 1(1), 2022, 33-39

[30]. E Ghaibi, et al., Comparison of Organizational Citizenship Behavior and Job Creativity between Male and Men's Education Personnel 1 Ahwaz, Eurasian Journal of Chemical, Medicinal and Petroleum Research, 1(2), 2022, 49-57

[31]. F Afkar, S Golalipour, M Akanchi, SM Sajedi, A Zandi Qashghaie, Systematic Reviews of Different Types of Drug Delivery in the Treatment and Prevention of Oral and Dental and Cardiorespiratory Diseases in Patients and Animals Involved, NeuroQuantology, 2022, 20 (8), 632-642

[32]. F Atashzadeh-Shoorideh, S Parvizy, M Hosseini, Y Raziani,et al., Developing and validating the nursing presence scale for hospitalized patients, BMC nursing, 2022, 21 (1), 1-16

[33]. F Karimzadeh, et al., Comparative evaluation of bacterial colonization on removable dental prostheses in patients with COVID-19: A clinical study, The Journal of Prosthetic Dentistry, 2021, 1-3

[34]. F Mirakhori, M Moafi, M Milanifard, A Asadi rizi, H Tahernia, Diagnosis and Treatment Methods in Alzheimer's Patients Based on Modern Techniques: The Orginal Article, Journal of Pharmaceutical Negative Results, 2022, 13 (1), 1889-1907

[35]. F Najafi, et al., The Relationship between General Health and Quality of Work Life of Nurses Working in Zahedan Teaching Hospitals. Iranian J of Rehabilitation Research in Nursing 2018; 4 (2): 53-9.

[36]. H Ashayeri, R Mohseni, Z Khazaie, S Golalipour, ZA Bondarabadi, Systematic Investigation of the Occurrence of Dental Problems, Cardiopulmonary Injuries and Duration of Hospitalization in ICU in Patients Affected by Covid-19 and Intubation in them, Tobacco Regulatory Science (TRS), 2022, 2124-2146

[37]. H Danesh, A Bahmani, F Moradi, B Shirazipour, M Milani Fard, Pharmacological Evaluation of Covid 19 Vaccine in Acute and Chronic Inflammatory Neuropathies, Journal of Medicinal and Chemical Sciences, 5(4), 2022, 561-570

[38]. H Daneste; A Sadeghzadeh; M Mokhtari; H Mohammadkhani; F Lavaee; J Moayedi; Immunoexpression of p53 mutant-type in Iranian patients with primary and recurrence oral squamous cell carcinoma. European Journal of Translational Myology, 2022

[39]. H Jahandideh, A Yarahmadi, S Rajaieh, AO Shirazi, M Milanifard, et al., Cone-beam computed tomography guidance in functional endoscopic sinus surgery: a retrospective cohort study, J Pharm Ree Int, 2020, 31 (6), 1-7

[40]. H Kalantari, et al., Determination of COVID-19 prevalence with regards to age range of patients referring to the hospitals located in western Tehran, Iran. Gene reports. 2020;21: 100910.

[41]. H Mirfakhraee, S Golalipour, F Ensafi, A Ensafi, S Hajisadeghi, Survival rate of Maxillary and Mandibular Implants used to Support Complete-arch Fixed Prostheses & Investigation of internal and Neurological manifestations, NeuroQuantology, 2022, 20 (6), 5118-5126

[42]. H Mirjalili, H Amani, A Ismaili, MM Fard, A Abdolrazaghnejad, Evaluation of Drug Therapy in Non-Communicable Diseases; a Review Study, Journal of Medicinal and Chemical Sciences, 2022, 5 (2), 204-214

[43]. H Tahernia, et al., Diagnosis and Treatment of MS in Patients Suffering from Various Degrees of the Disease with a Clinical Approach: The Original Article, Journal of Pharmaceutical Negative Results, 2022, 13 (1), 1908-1921

[44]. I Karampela, M Dalamaga, Could Respiratory Fluoroquinolones, Levofloxacin and Moxifloxacin, prove to be Beneficial as an Adjunct Treatment in COVID-19? Archives of medical research. 2020;51(7):741-2.

[45]. I Seifi, D Shojaei, SJ Barbin, A Bahmani, Z Seraj, Methods of Diagnosis and Treatment of MS Disease Based on a Clinical Trial: The Original Article, Tobacco Regulatory Science (TRS),2022, 2351-2384

[46]. JP Montani, Vliet VB. General physiology and pathophysiology of the renin-angiotensin system. Angiotensin Vol. I: Springer; 2004: 3-29.

[47]. K Goyal, et al., Fear of COVID 2019: First suicidal case in India! Asian J of psychiatry 2020; 49: 101989.

[48]. L Sadati, A Askarkhah, S Hannani, M Moazamfard, M Abedinzade, PM Alinejad, N Saraf, A Arabkhazaei, Assessment of staff performance in cssd unit by 360-degree evaluation method, Asia Pacific Journal of Health Management, 2020, 15(4), 71-77

[49]. L Sadati, ZN Khanegah, NS Shahri, F Edalat, Postoperative pain experienced by the candidates for gynecological surgery with lithotomy position, Iranian Journal of Obstetrics, Gynecology and Infertility, 2022, 24(12), 29-34

[50]. M Aminzadeh, et al., The Frequency of Medication Errors and Factors Influencing the Lack of Reporting Medication Errors in Nursing at Teaching Hospital of Qazvin University of Medical Sciences, 2012. J of Health 2015; 6 (2): 169-79.

[51]. M Barzideh, A Choobineh, Tabatabaei S. Job stress dimensions and their relationship to general health status in nurses. Occupational Medicine 2012; 4 (3): 17-27.

[52]. M Milanifard, G Hassanzadeha, Anthropometric study of nasal index in Hausa ethnic population of northwestern Nigeria, J Contemp Med Sci|, 2018, 4 (1), 26-29

[53]. M Mileski, et al., The impact of nurse practitioners on hospitalizations and discharges from long-term nursing facilities: a systematic review. Healthcare 2020; 8 (2): 114-34.

[54]. MGS Borba, et al. Effect of high vs low doses of chloroquine diphosphate as adjunctive therapy for patients hospitalized with severe acute respiratory syndrome coronavirus 2 (SARS-CoV-2) infection: a randomized clinical trial. JAMA network open. 2020;3(4): e208857-e.

[55]. MJ Gadlage, et al., Murine hepatitis virus nonstructural protein 4 regulates virus-induced membrane modifications and replication complex function. J Virol, 2010. 84(1): p. 280-90.

[56]. MM Fard, Effects of Micronutrients in Improving Fatigue, Weakness and Irritability, GMJ Med. 2021, 5 (1): 391 395

[57]. MR Moghadam, A Shams, ZS Moosavifard, F Shahnazari, D Shojaei, Principles of Health Care for Patients Involved in Fracture, Multiple Trauma and Type of Burns in Operating Room & Intensive Care Unit: The Original Article, Tobacco Regulatory Science (TRS), 2022, 2839-2854

[58]. N Alrabadi, et al. Medication errors: a focus on nursing practice. J of Pharmaceutical Health Services Research 2021; 12 (1): 78-86.

[59]. N Asadi, et al., Investigating the Relationship Between Corona Anxiety and Nursing Care Behaviors Working in Coronary Referral Hospitals. IJPCP 2020; 26 (3): 306-19.

[60]. N Shahkarami, M Nazari, M Milanifard, R Tavakolimoghadam, A Bahmani, The assessment of iron deficiency biomarkers in both anemic and non-anemic dialysis patients: A systematic review and meta-analysis, Eurasian Chemical Communications 4 (6), 463-472

[61]. N Zaimzadeh, et al., Comparison of vitamin D dietary intake among four phenotypes of polycystic ovary syndrome and its association with serum androgenic components, Razi Journal of Medical Sciences, 2018, 25 (2), 87

[62]. N Zaimzadeh, et al., The study of dietary intake of micronutrients in four phenotypes of polycystic ovary syndrome separately based on Rotterdam criteria, Razi Journal of Medical Sciences, 2018, 25 (3), 59-68

[63]. S Azizi Aram, S Bashar poor, The role of rumination, emotion regulation and responsiveness to stress in predicting of Corona anxiety (COVID-19) among nurses. Quarterly J of Nursing Management 2020; 9 (3): 8-18.

[64]. S Ghorbanizadeh, Y Raziani, M Amraei, M Heydarian, Care and precautions in performing CT Scans in children, Journal of Pharmaceutical Negative Results, 2021, 12 (1), 54

[65]. S Golalipour, et al., Examination of Dental Problems and Radiological and Cardiac Evaluations in Patients Affected by Covid-19, NeuroQuantology, 2022, 20 (8), 1519- 1527

[66]. S Hariri, S Golalipour, et al., Examining the Fracture Strength of Implant-based Fixed Partial Prostheses with Different Dimensions of Connectors in the System CAM/CAD/Zir, Tobacco Regulatory Science (TRS), 2022, 2310-2329

[67]. S Mahmoodi, et al., General health and related factors in employed nurses in Medical-Educational Centers in Rasht. JHNM 2015; 25 (1): 63-72.

[68]. S Musaei, The Effect of Pregnancy on the Skin, Eurasian Journal of Chemical, Medicinal and Petroleum Research, 2023, 2 (1), 17-23

[69]. S Sheikh, F Hatami, D Shojaei, A Shams, R Sourani, The Principles Of Treatment Staff Care Of Elderly Patients Under Burn & Plastic Surgery And With Covid-19 In ICU & Operating Room Based On Clinical Points: The Original Article, Journal of Pharmaceutical Negative Results, 2022 1967

[70]. S.H Salehi, K As'adi, S.J Mousavi, S Shoar, Evaluation of Amniotic Membrane Effectiveness in Skin Graft Donor Site Dressing in Burn Patients, Indian J Surg, 2015 Dec;77(Suppl 2):427-31.

[71]. S.H Salehi, M.J Fatemih, K Aśadi, S Shoar, A Der Ghazarian, R Samimi, Electrical injury in construction workers: a special focus on injury with electrical power, Burns, 2014 Mar;40(2):300-4.

[72]. SE Ahmadi, M Farzanehpour, AMM Fard, MM Fard, HEG Ghaleh, Succinct review on biological and clinical aspects of Coronavirus disease 2019 (COVID-19), Romanian Journal of Military Medicine, 2022, 356-365

[73]. SZ Nazardani, et al., A comprehensive evaluation of the Sports Physiotherapy curriculum. Eurasian Journal of Chemical, Medicinal and Petroleum Research, 2(1), 2023, 10-16

[74]. TSH Abadi, et al., Depression, stress and anxiety of nurses in COVID-19 pandemic in Nohe-Dey Hospital in Torbat-e-Heydariyeh city, Iran. J of Military Med 2020; 22 (6): 526-33.

[75]. Y Raziani, BS Othman, Ointment therapy and prevention of cannulation-induced superficial phlebitis, Veins and Lymphatics, 2021, 10 (2)

[76]. Y Raziani, et al., Pistacia atlantica as an effective remedy for diabetes: a randomised, double-blind, placebo-controlled trial, Australian Journal of Herbal and Naturopathic Medicine, 2022, 34(3), 118-124.

[77]. Y Raziani, S Raziani, Evaluation of Mental Health of Chemotherapy-Treated Cancer Nurses, Journal of Medicinal and Chemical Sciences, 2021, 4(4), 351-363.

[78]. Y Raziani, S Raziani, The effect of air pollution on myocardial infarction, Journal of Chemical Reviews, 2021, 3(1), 83-96.

[79]. Y. Raziani, et al., A common but unknown disease; A case series study, Annals of Medicine and Surgery, 2021, 69, 102739.

[80]. YA Helmy, et al., The COVID-19 pandemic: a comprehensive review of taxonomy, genetics, epidemiology, diagnosis, treatment, and control. Journal of Clinical Medicine. 2020;9(4):1225.

[81]. Z Khezerlou, D Shojaei, S Jafari, A Arabkhazaie, SHA Abadi, The Principles of Care of the Treatment Staff for the Elderly with Fracture Problems and Corona Virus in the Special Care Unit, Tobacco Regulatory Science (TRS), 2022, 2825-2838

[82]. Z Malekpour-Dehkordi, M Nourbakhsh, M Shahidi, N Sarraf, R Sharifi. Silymarin diminishes oleic acid-induced lipid accumulation in HepG2 cells by modulating the expression of endoplasmic reticulum stress markers. *Journal of Herbal Medicine*. 2022; 33:100565.

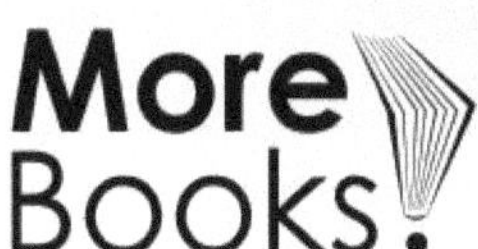

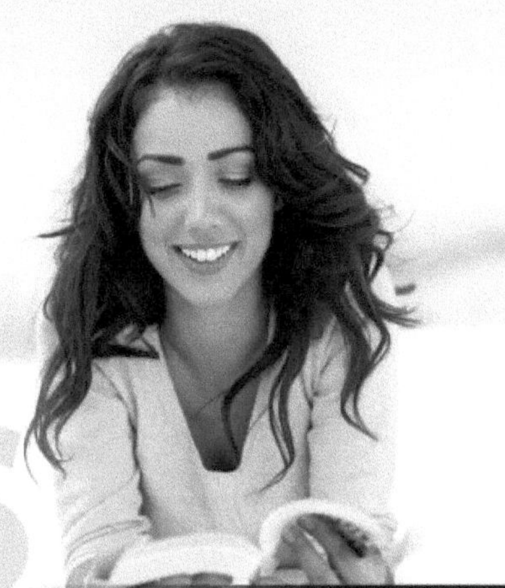

yes
I want morebooks!

Buy your books fast and straightforward online - at one of world's fastest growing online book stores! Environmentally sound due to Print-on-Demand technologies.

Buy your books online at
www.morebooks.shop

Kaufen Sie Ihre Bücher schnell und unkompliziert online – auf einer der am schnellsten wachsenden Buchhandelsplattformen weltweit! Dank Print-On-Demand umwelt- und ressourcenschonend produziert.

Bücher schneller online kaufen
www.morebooks.shop

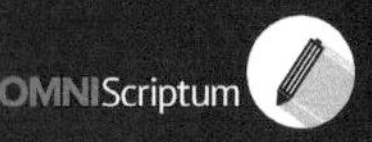

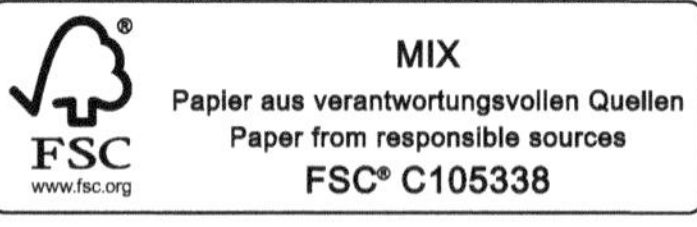

Printed by Books on Demand GmbH, Norderstedt / Germany